PROCEDURES
in CRITICAL
CARE

Notice

Medicine is an ever-changing science. As new research and clinical experience broaden our knowledge, changes in treatment and drug therapy are required. The authors and the publisher of this work have checked with sources believed to be reliable in their efforts to provide information that is complete and generally in accord with the standards accepted at the time of publication. However, in view of the possibility of human error or changes in medical sciences, neither the authors nor the publisher nor any other party who has been involved in the preparation or publication of this work warrants that the information contained herein is in every respect accurate or complete, and they disclaim all responsibility for any errors or omissions or for the results obtained from use of the information contained in this work. Readers are encouraged to confirm the information contained herein with other sources. For example and in particular, readers are advised to check the product information sheet included in the package of each drug they plan to administer to be certain that the information contained in this work is accurate and that changes have not been made in the recommended dose or in the contraindications for administration. This recommendation is of particular importance in connection with new or infrequently used drugs.

PROCEDURES *in* CRITICAL CARE

C. William Hanson III, MD

Professor of Anesthesiology and Critical Care, Surgery
 and Internal Medicine
Section Chief, Critical Care Medicine
Medical Director, Surgical Intensive Care Unit
Medical Director, ICU Telemedicine
Department of Anesthesiology and Critical Care
University of Pennsylvania Health System
Philadelphia, Pennsylvania

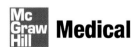 **Medical**

New York Chicago San Francisco Lisbon London Madrid Mexico City
Milan New Delhi San Juan Seoul Singapore Sydney Toronto

Procedures in Critical Care

1 2 3 4 5 6 7 8 9   CTP/CTP   12 11 10 9 8

Set ISBN 978-0-07-148181-6
Set MHID 0-07-148181-8
Book ISBN 978-0-07-160520-5
Book MHID 0-07-160520-7
DVD ISBN 978-0-07-160521-2
DVD MHID 0-07-160521-5

This book was set in Cheltenham by International Typesetting and Composition.
The editors were Ruth Weinberg and Christie Naglieri.
The production supervisor was Sherri Souffrance.
Project management was provided by Vastavikta Sharma, International Typesetting and Composition.
The designer was Eve Siegel.
Credit: Simon Fraser/RVI, Newcastle upon Tyne / Photo Researchers, Inc.
Caption: Sampling of cerebrospinal fluid.
Cover Designer: Mary McKeon.
China Translation & Printing, Ltd., was printer and binder.

This book is printed on acid-free paper.

Library of Congress Cataloging-in-Publication Data

Hanson, C. William (Clarence William), 1955
    Procedures in critical care / C. William Hanson III.—1st ed.
        p. ; cm.
    Includes bibliographical references and index.
    ISBN-13: 978-0-07-148181-6 (hardcover : alk. paper)
    ISBN-10: 0-07-148181-8 (hardcover : alk. paper)
    1. Critical care medicine.   I. Title.
    [DNLM: 1. Intensive Care—methods. WX 218 H251p   2009]
    RC86.7.H368   2009
    616.02′8—dc22
                                                    2008006225

*This text is dedicated to the residents, fellows, and
fellow intensivists with whom it has been my privilege
to work over the past 25 years both at Stanford
University and the University of Pennsylvania.*

Contents

SECTION IV: CARDIOVASCULAR PROCEDURES

SECTION V: GASTROINTESTINAL FEATURES

SECTION VI: GENITOURINARY PROCEDURES

SECTION VII: EXTREMITY PROCEDURES

Preface

Today's intensive care unit is a technologically rich environment where skilled teams employ advanced treatments to monitor and support organ systems in patients with medical illnesses, following traumatic injuries, or after surgery. While the invasive procedures undertaken in the intensive care unit (ICU) may come with benefits, they often come with risks, including those of infection, bleeding, procedural errors, and device failure. For a variety of reasons, including increasing specialization, workforce turnover, and constrained training hours, it is not uncommon for nursing and medical practitioners to have limited exposure to advanced critical care procedures. This book was designed to illustrate the fundamentals of a broad variety of techniques organized by organ system, and to thereby serve as an introduction to critical care interventions. Each procedure chapter consists of an introduction, definitions and terms, techniques, pearls and pitfalls, as well as a series of illustrative line art and photographs. The book is designed for students, novice practitioners, and experts who want exposure to procedures outside of their general field of expertise. In addition to the printed material, a DVD containing narrated video segments depicting procedures commonly performed in the ICU has been included as part of the book.

C. William Hanson III, MD

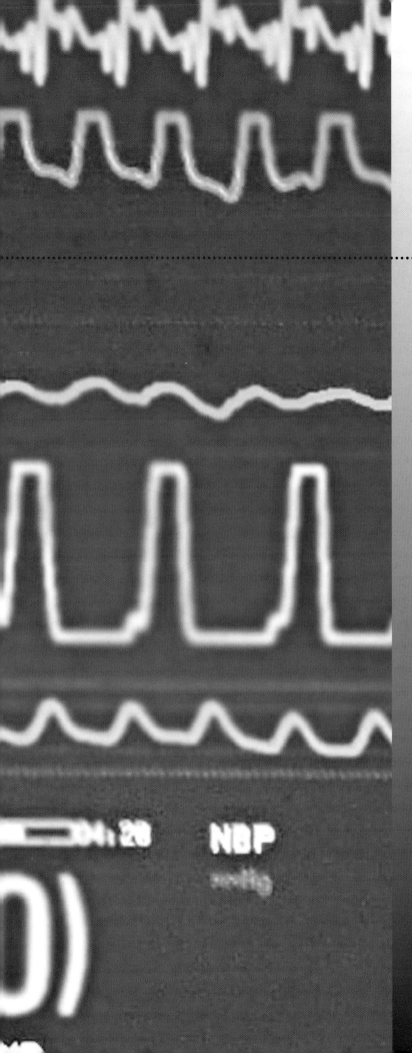

SECTION I

ICU
Basics

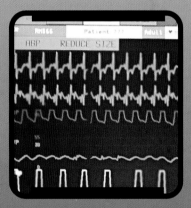

CHAPTER 1

The ICU Room and Equipment

Introduction

The intensive care unit (ICU) room is a highly specialized environment, differing in many ways from a standard hospital room. ICU rooms are staffed with a higher nursing staffing ratio, typically one nurse to two rooms, and a premium is placed on patient visibility. Units are often constructed in such a manner that all patients can be under continuous observation from the central-nursing station, either directly or using cameras. Patients are individually monitored with a variety of bedside physiologic monitors, and ICU rooms are designed to have redundant gas and electric sources.

Definitions and Terms

- Headwall: The wall behind the head of a patient in an ICU, in which electrical, gas, and equipment mounts are deployed—while headwalls are typical, columns and movable, jointed arms are used in some units (ie, pediatric) to permit more flexible bed/crib configurations (Figure 1-1).

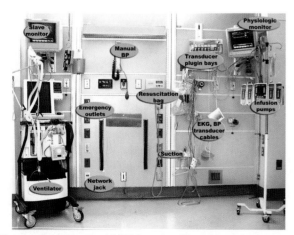

Figure 1-1. Typical ICU headwall with various components and utilities.

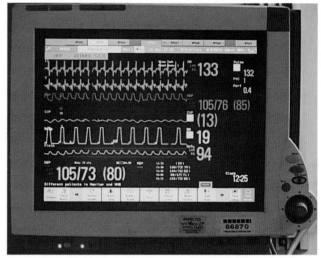

Figure 1-2. Physiologic monitor which display patient data in a central location as waveforms and numeric readouts.

- Physiologic monitor: A piece of medical equipment that serves as a central aggregation and display location for many medically significant physiologic variables, including electrocardiogram (ECG), various pressure waveforms, noninvasive blood pressure, pulse oximetry, respiration, temperature, and so on (Figure 1-2).

- Telemetry: Electronic transmission of medical data to a central analysis station (Figure 1-3).

- Electrocardiography: Analysis and display of data regarding cardiac conduction and rhythm (Figure 1-4).

- Pulse oximetry: Photoelectric, noninvasive measurement of capillary oxygen levels using light transmission through a capillary bed to a receiver (Figure 1-5).

- Impedance pneumography: A technique by which respiratory rate is measured using electrical changes between ECG leads induced by changes in intrathoracic air volume during inspiration and expiration.

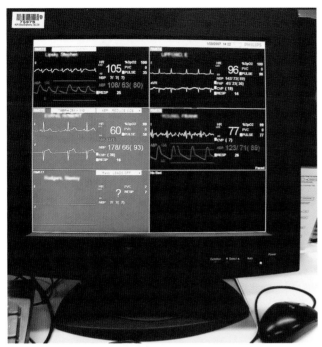

Figure 1-3. Central monitor on a nursing unit, where the key data from all of the patients on a unit are aggregated, and from which alarms are generated to all providers on a unit.

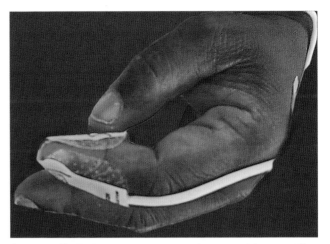

Figure 1-5. Pulse oximeter on a finger, with transillumination of the finger by light of a specific wavelength.

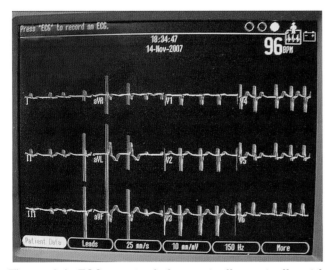

Figure 1-4. ECG acquired electronically, typically with preliminary automated analysis, which is then printed for the medical record.

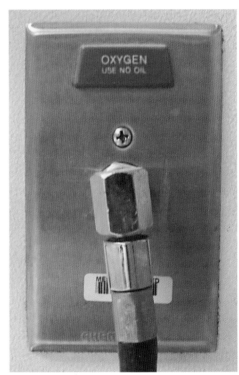

Figure 1-6. Wall oxygen source, which is color-coded green (in the United States) and specifically fitted for oxygen connectors and tubing.

- Wall oxygen supply: Oxygen is piped into hospitals from a central supply source typically on the hospital grounds—gases are distributed to outlets throughout the hospital which are both color coded and distributed using gas specific connectors to mechanical ventilators and/or gas blenders. While colors for medical gases vary among countries, green (Figure 1-6) is used to indicate oxygen in the United States (whereas white is used in the United Kingdom). Wall oxygen is supplied at 50 pounds per square inch (psi) and distributed throughout the hospital from central liquid oxygen containers.

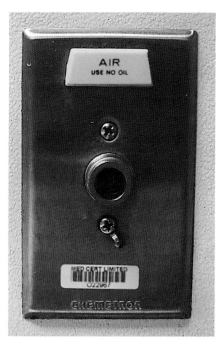

Figure 1-7. Wall air source, which is specifically color-coded yellow (in the United States) and specifically fitted for air (as distinct from oxygen) connectors and tubing.

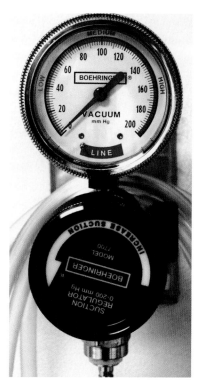

Figure 1-8. Wall suction, which is adjustable with an adjustable regulator. Suction tubing is color coded and fitted distinctly from air and oxygen fittings.

■ Wall air supply: Compressed air is piped to ICU headwalls using a separate and distinct piping system and is dispensed at the bedside through a specific color coded and connector specific gas outlet—air is blended with oxygen to dispense specific oxygen concentrations to the patient. In the United States, the color yellow (Figure 1-7) is used to indicate compressed air (whereas black and white are used in the United Kingdom). Wall air is typically supplied at 50 psi.

■ Wall suction: A separate suction system is available at each ICU bedside and used for a variety of applications (Figure 1-8), including suction on drains (ie, chest tubes, gastric tubes, abdominal drains, etc.) and pulmonary secretion removal. Vacuum pressure is, approximately, 10 psi, and, as with medical gases, vacuum lines have specific connectors and are colored white in the United States (whereas they are yellow in the United Kingdom)

■ Emergency power system: An electrical supply system in a hospital that is automatically set to convert to generator power in the event of loss of external electrical supply to a hospital—emergency outlets are red (Figure 1-9) to distinguish them from regular outlets (Figure 1-10).

■ ICU rooms are often equipped with an emergency call button (Figure 1-11).

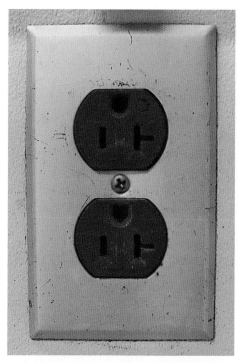

Figure 1-9. Emergency power supply outlet, which is color-coded red, and provides power attached to the backup electrical generator, which supplies power in the event of an interruption of supply from the utility company.

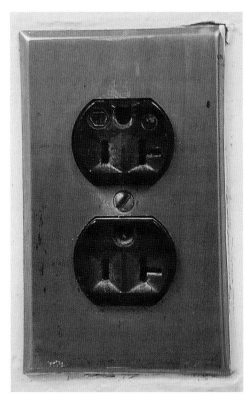

Figure 1-10. Standard power outlet.

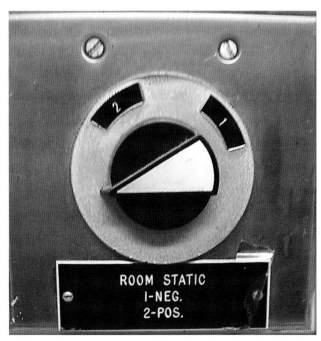

Figure 1-12. Room pressure regulator, which raises or lowers ICU room atmospheric pressure relative to the pressure outside of the room—used to partition the air in the room from the rest of the unit.

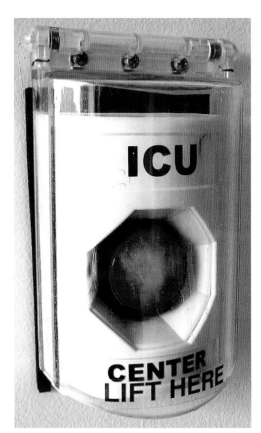

Figure 1-11. Emergency bedside "code" button which may be used to summon help in the event of an emergency.

- ICU room pressure may be adjustable to allow keep air outside of the room from coming in (positive pressure) in, for example, patients at risk for nosocomial infections, or to prevent air inside the room from leaving (negative pressure) in, for example, patients with highly contagious airborne organisms (Figure 1-12).
- Transducer: A device for converting energy from one form to another, typically a pressure wave to an electronic signal in the ICU, where fluid waves are measured and displayed (Figure 1-13).
- Infusion pump: A device that controls the administration of medications or fluids (Figure 1-14).

 Techniques

- Standard vital signs in an ICU
  - Continuous electrocardiography using one or more leads, typically leads II and V_5 (lead II is preferred for arrhythmia analysis because it is best for showing the P wave, whereas V_5 is preferred to detect ischemia).
  - Blood pressure using noninvasive or continuous intra-arterial measurement (Figure 1-15).
  - Pulse oximetry in patients receiving supplemental oxygen.

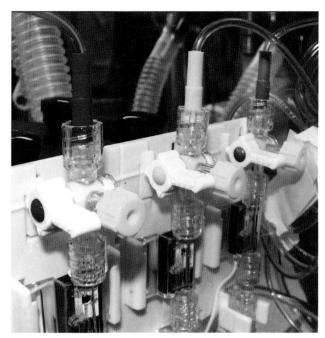

Figure 1-13. Electronic transducer which converts fluid pressures and waveforms into an electrical signal that is interpretable by bedside physiologic monitor.

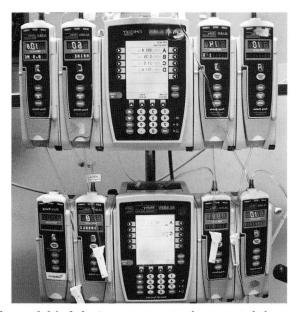

Figure 1-14. Infusion pumps, used to control the rate of delivery of fluids or medications to a patient, and prevent infusion of air or debris.

—Respiratory rate using impedance pneumography.

—Temperature can be measured intermittently (Figure 1-16) or continuously through indwelling devices such as the pulmonary artery catheter or a thermistor-equipped urinary catheter.

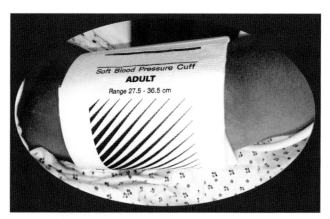

Figure 1-15. Disposable blood pressure cuff for automated measurement.

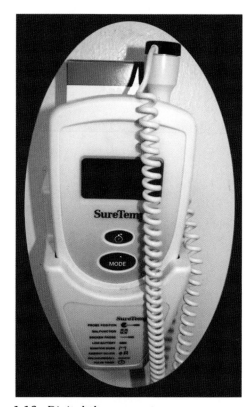

Figure 1-16. Digital thermometer.

■Additional discretionary ICU monitoring

—Automatic, continuous arrhythmia detection may be indicated in certain patient populations at high risk for rhythm abnormalities (Figure 1-17).

—Fluid waveform and pressure are used to analyze intravascular and other intracompartmental pressure (ie, pulmonary artery, cerebrospinal fluid [CSF]) in patients undergoing advanced monitoring.

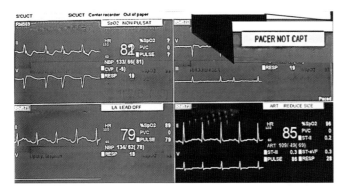

Figure 1-17. Central nursing unit monitor with automated rhythm detection.

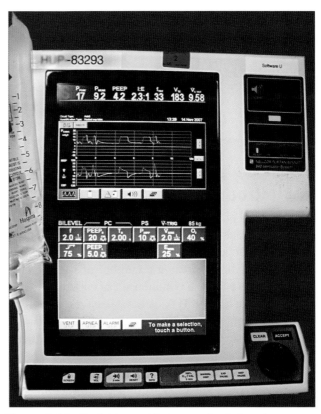

Figure 1-19. Bedside ventilator readout showing a variety of ventilator settings and patient measurements.

—Tissue and blood oxygen saturation may be displayed continuously from a variety of sources including central vascular sites (ie, mixed venous oxygen saturation), brain (ie, cerebral oximetry).

—Intermittent or continuous cardiac output can be displayed on dedicated bedside devices or through a suitably interfaced physiologic monitoring system (Figure 1-18).

—A variety of respiratory parameters can be measured through a mechanical ventilator in a mechanically ventilated patient, including respiratory rate, tidal volume, minute ventilation, compliance, autopeep, and so on (Figure 1-19).

 Suggested Reading

Guidelines/Practice Parameters Committee of the American College of Critical Care Medicine, Society of Critical Care Medicine. Guidelines for intensive care unit design. *Cri Care Med.* 1995;23:582–88.

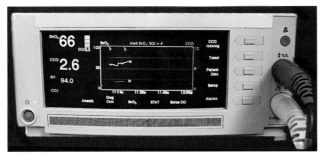

Figure 1-18. Physiologic monitor dedicated to the display of cardiac output and central vascular oxygen saturation—these data may also be sent directly to the main bedside physiologic monitor.

CHAPTER 2

The ICU Bed

Introduction

Intensive care unit (ICU) patients can develop a variety of complications related to prolonged immobilization and recumbent positioning while in the ICU, and, increasingly, obese patients present a number of specific challenges. ICU beds have a common set of capabilities, and a variety of specialty ICU beds have been developed for specific patient populations (Figure 2-1) including patients at risk for decubitus ulcers, obese patients, patients with fractures. A standard ICU bed typically has electric and manual controls, side rails, wheels and a brake, a removable headboard to allow procedures (ie, endotracheal intubation, vascular access) from the head of the bed, and intravenous (IV) pole mounts.

Definitions and Terms

- Trendelenburg position: Bed position in which the head is lower than the feet—typically used to increase venous return to the heart in hypovolemic shock or to distend blood vessels superior to the heart during venous access procedures (Figure 2-2).

- Reverse Trendelenburg position: Used in the ICU to elevate the head above the heart to diminish venous return, or to decrease the likelihood of passive regurgitation of gastric contents in patient in whom leg flexion is contraindicated (ie, following femoral arterial cannulation).

- Elevated head of bed (also known as Fowler or semi-Fowler position): Standard nursing position in an ICU patient, where not otherwise contraindicated—used as one element of the "bundle" of interventions designed to reduce the incidence of ventilator associated pneumonia, by lowering the risk of passive aspiration of gastric contents (Figure 2-3).

- Decubitus ulcer: Skin ulceration caused by prolonged pressure on a vulnerable area (ie, sacrum, occiput), typically in a bed-ridden patient.

- Rotation therapy: An approach to the prevention of pulmonary complications and decubitus ulcers by continuously rotating the entire patient.

- Percussion therapy: An approach to the prevention of ICU complications by continuous bed vibration intended to facilitate the mobilization of pulmonary secretions.

- Pressure relief therapy: A variety of approaches to the redistribution of weight away from vulnerable pressure points—designed to prevent or treat decubitus ulcers (Figure 2-4).

Techniques

- A standard ICU bed is suitable for the care of most ICU patients and may be equipped with a pressure relief mattress designed to prevent the formation of decubitus ulcers.

- A bariatric bed is designed to accommodate and facilitate the care of the obese patient, having a larger surface area and greater hydraulic lifting power.

- A fall prevention bed can be lowered to the floor to limit the potential of injury in patients at risk for falls.

- Pressure relief beds may include automatic patient rotation, air/fluid mattress technology.

- A kinetic therapy bed allows the patient with adult respiratory distress syndrome (ARDS) and/or spinal cord injury to undergo continuous rotation and percussion to facilitate secretion mobilization and drainage without the need for manual mobilization of the patient.

Clinical Pearls and Pitfalls

- ICU specialty beds are expensive and specific indications should be developed for individual bed usage.

- The choice of specialty beds is usually made collaboratively between the physician and nursing members of the critical care time.

- Individual hospitals often have a resource person with specific expertise in specialty beds.

- The increasing number of obese patients in the healthcare system has led to the development of new technologies such as bed scales, specialty (ie, ceiling) lifts, and bariatric chairs for early mobilization of these patients.

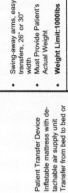
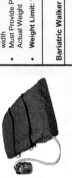

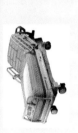
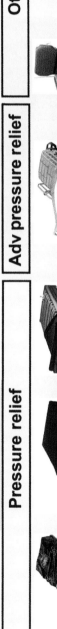

Vac ats

- Negative Pressure Wound Therapy
- Chronic open wounds
- Diabetic ulcers
- Acute and traumatic wounds
- Flaps and grafts
- Surgical wounds
- Partial thickness burns, and pressure ulcers.

Contraindications:
- Malignancy in the wound
- Untreated osteomyelitis
- Nonenteric and unexplored fistula
- Necrotic tissue with eschar present

Indications:
- Patients at high risk of pressure ulcers
- Management of Stage I, II, III and IV pressure ulcers

Contraindications:
- Unstable cervical, thoracic and/or lumbar fracture
- Cervical Traction

- **Weight limit: 350 Lbs**

**Do not place VAC dressing over exposed blood vessels or organs.

- **Vac ATS Accessories** ⟶

Item	Lawson #
Vac Canister	129259
1 Liter Canister	146636
Sml Dressing	129256
Med Dressing	129257
Lg Dressing	129258
X-Lg Dressing	129261
Ab Dressing	129262
White Foam	130109
T.R.A.C. Foam	130807
"Y" Connector	129260

Bariatric

- Built in scale
- Intellidrive power transport

Contraindications:
- Not for patient's with pressure ulcers
- Bariatric Patient's with pressure ulcers consult your Clinical Specialist

- **Weight limit: 500 lbs**

- Extra wide 42' bariatric Bed
- Built in scale
- IntelliDrive power transport
- Full Chair positioning
- Full Egress Position
- Retractable Foot

Contraindications:
- Not for patient's with pressure ulcers
- Bariatric Patient's with pressure ulcers consult your Clinical Specialist

- **Weight limit: 460 lbs**
- **Height limit: 7 feet**

- Expandable bariatric bed from 39", 48" or 54"
- Basic Mattress included

Accessories:
- Trapeze
- RS Bariatric

- **Weight limit: 1000 lbs**

Fall prevention

- Fall Prevention and risk mitigation
- Electric Hi-Lo bed
- Lock out functions
- Raised border mattress included
- Can Order second floor mat through Sun-rise

- **Weight Limit: 500 lbs**

Kinetic therapy

- Kinetic Therapy for the critically ill, immobilized patient
- Specifically for spinal injuries or ARDS patients

Indications:
- Treatment and prevention of pulmonary complications
- Thoracic or lumbar fracture
- Cervical Traction
- Skeletal Traction

Contraindications:
- Patients that do not tolerate rotation.

- **Weight limit: 500lbs**

Pressure relief

- Pressure relief overlay
- Anti shear layer

Indications:
- Patients at high risk of pressure ulcers

Contraindications:
- Unstable cervical, thoracic and/or lumbar fracture
- Cervical Traction

- **Weight Limit: 1000 lbs**

- Use on Care 1000 Beds.
- An Aggressive Therapeutic mattress
- Alternating pressure therapy with low air-loss
- Maximum inflate mode for immediate firm surface
- 1 in 3 alternating variable time cycles

- **Weight Limit: 350 lbs**

- Placed on Regular or HiLo Beds
- An Aggressive Therapeutic mattress
- Alternating pressure therapy with low air-loss
- Maximum inflate mode for immediate firm surface
- 1 in 3 alternating variable time cycles

- **Weight Limit: 350 lbs**

Adv pressure relief

- Air Fluidized Therapy Unit
- Provides combination of air fluidized therapy and low air loss therapy
- Prevention/treatment to Stage IV pressure ulcers.
- When mobility and HOB elevation is the goal of therapy
- Post op flap and graft surgery.

Contraindications:
- Unstable spinal cord injuries, long bone traction

- **Weight limit: 350 lbs**

Other

- Bariatric Mobile Chair Recliner
- Switches from full seat to supine position
- Side rails raise or lower for transfer or safety

- **Weight Limits: 850lbs**
- Must Provide Patient's Actual Weight
- Models:
  - 400lbs - 24" seat width
  - 600lbs - 27" seat width
  - 850lbs - 31" seat width

- Patient Transfer Device
- Inflatable mattress with detachable air supply unit
- Transfer from bed to bed or bed to litter
- Can remain un-inflated under the patient
- Models: 34", 39", and 50" mattresses

- **Weight Limit: 900lbs**
- Must Provide Patient's Actual Weight

Figure 2-1. Chart of various specialty beds with applications, costs, and additional details. *Copyright Trustees of the University of Pennsylvania, with permission.*

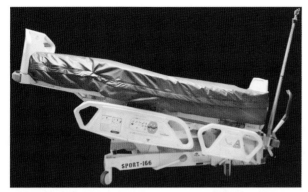

Figure 2-2. ICU bed with pressure relief mattress and standard controls in Trendelenburg (head down) position.

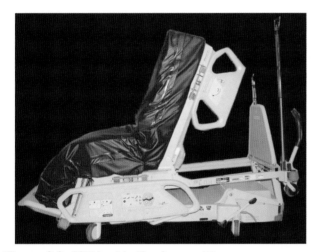

Figure 2-3. ICU bed in Fowler position.

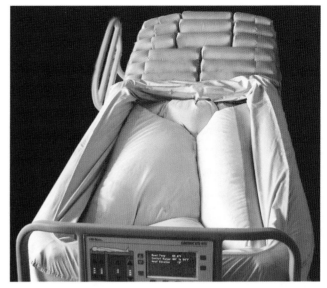

Figure 2-4. Specialty pressure relief air/fluid mattress, in which warmed air passes continuously through beads and the mattress surface, minimizing local skin pressure.

Suggested Reading

Gebhardt KS, Bliss MR, Winright PL, Thomas J. Pressure relieving supports in ICU. *J Wound Care.* 1996;5:116–121.

Ryan DW. The fluidized bed. *Intensive Care Med.* 1995;21:270–276.

CHAPTER 3

The Universal Protocol in the ICU

Introduction

The universal protocol was designed to prevent wrong site, wrong procedure, and wrong person surgery and has evolved from collaboration among accreditation organizations and professional societies. It was introduced as a standard in 2004.

Definitions and Terms

The protocol is a three-step process including (1) preprocedure identification and verification, (2) site marking, and (3) performance of a "time-out" prior to initiation of the procedure. A mnemonic is "Correct Person, Correct Procedure, and Correct Site."

Techniques

- Indications in the ICU

  —Surgical/invasive procedures falling within the scope of universal protocol guidelines include, but are not limited to, cardioversions, cardiac and vascular catheterizations (ie, pulmonary artery catheter placement and vasculare cannulation), transesophageal echocardiography, endoscopies, thoracentesis, chest tube insertions, paracentesis, lumbar puncture, incisions and drainage of wounds, and so on.

- Preprocedure patient identification elements

  —Patient name and date of birth

  —Medical record number

  —Verbal identification with patient and/or family member

- Preprocedure verification (Figure 3-1)

  —Procedure confirmation with patient or family/designee

  —Consent obtained for procedure

  —Relevant documentation performed

  —Indications for procedure

- Site marking (Figure 3-2)

  —Marking of the site is required for procedures involving left/right distinction, multiple structures (ie, fingers and toes) or multiple levels (ie, spinal levels).

  —Site marking is not required for interventional procedures for which the site is not predetermined, such as arterial line placement, or when procedure is performed under urgent or emergency conditions.

Universal Protocol			
Patient identification (need 2): ☐ Name/DOB ☐ Verbal with patient and/or family ☐ Other (MRN)-Use when there are 2 patients with same name and DOB	**Procedure verification:** ☐ Procedure confirmed with patient or family/designee ☐ Consent for procedure signed ☐ Relevant documentation completed, reviewed and signed ☐ Clinical indications for procedure	**Site marked (operative site):** ☐ Yes ☐ N/A	**Time-out with all members of procedure team immediately prior to procedure:** ☐ Correct patient identified ☐ Agreement on procedure ☐ Correct side and site ☐ N/A ☐ Correct patient position ☐ Availability of correct implant/equip. ☐ N/A
Completed by: Name (Print) _____ Signature _____ Date _____ Time_____			

Figure 3-1. A sample universal protocol checklist.

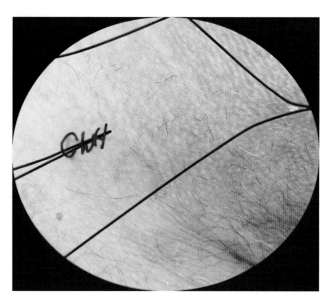

Figure 3-2. Example of site marking with operator's initials at the site of left internal jugular, as viewed from the left side of patient's neck.

—Marking should be unambiguous (ie, use initials of operator or YES).

—Marking should be made with ink that remains visible after skin preprocedure.

—Marking should remain visible after draping.

■ Time-out elements checked with all members of procedure team immediately prior to performance of procedure

—Verify correct patient identified

—Ensure agreement on planned procedure

—Verify correct side and site

—Verify correct patient position for procedure

—Ensure availability of all required equipment

 Clinical Pearls and Pitfalls

■ Marking a site with an X is ambiguous—this could be interpreted as "this *is* the site" or "this is *not* the site."

■ Certain sites (ie, teeth) need not be marked directly, but radiographs should be marked correctly.

■ Single organ sites need not necessarily be marked (ie, cardiac surgery, caesarian section).

 Suggested Reading

The Joint Commission. Universal protocol. http://www.jointcommission.org/PatientSafety/UniversalProtocol. (Accessed on May 11, 2008.)

CHAPTER 4

Hand Washing in the ICU

 ## Introduction

Hand washing has been shown to reduce nosocomial infection dating back to Semmelweis' historic research on obstetric infections in the 1800s. Hand washing is now the focus of recommendations and requirements from the Centers for Disease Control and the Joint Commission for Accreditation of Healthcare Organizations. It is also widely felt to be the best measure to prevent the emergence and transmission of drug-resistant nosocomial infections, such as Methicillin Resistant Staphylococcus Aureus (MRSA).

 ## Definitions and Terms

- Plain (detergent) soaps: Used for cleansing but lack intrinsic antimicrobial properties.

- Antimicrobial soaps Detergent plus an antimicrobial such as alcohol, chlorhexidine, or povidone-iodine.

- Alcohol-based hand rub: Contain ethanol or isopropanol and denature proteins when used in water-containing solutions; rapidly active against bacteria, mycobacteria, fungi, and viruses; typically combined with moisturizer to prevent hand chapping.

- Chlorhexidine and iodophors: Alternative antiseptic agents with intermediate speed of action and variable activity against infectious agents, chlorhexidine has good persistence (see below).

- Visibly soiled hands: Show visible dirt or proteinaceous material, blood, or body fluids.

- Persistent (antimicrobial) activity: The property of certain hand-cleansing agents having extended antimicrobial action.

 ## Techniques

- Visibly soiled hands: Wash with soap and water.

- Before eating or after using the restroom: Wash with soap and water.

- Not visibly soiled hands: Use an alcohol-based hand rub under the following circumstances:

  —Before direct patient contact

  —Before donning sterile gloves for a procedure

  —Before insertion of urinary catheters, intravascular devices, or other invasive devices

  —After contact with a patient's skin

  —After contact with bodily fluids, excretions, or dressings

  —After contact with inanimate objects in the immediate vicinity of a patient (ie, ventilator, bed rail)

  —After removing gloves

- Remove visible debris from beneath fingernails.

- Routine hand washing: Wet hands with water, apply recommended amount of soap, and rub hands together vigorously for at least 15 seconds covering all surfaces of hands and fingers. Dry with disposable paper towel and turn water off with towel.

- Decontamination with alcohol-based hand rub: Apply product to palm of one hand and rub hands together covering all surfaces of hands and fingers until hands are dry (Figure 4-1).

- Additional recommendations for healthcare workers

  —Remove rings, watches, and bracelets before hand scrub.

  —Do not wear artificial fingernails.

  —Keep natural fingernail length less than $1/4$ in long.

  —Wear gloves when in contact with blood or other infectious agents.

  —Remove gloves after patient care.

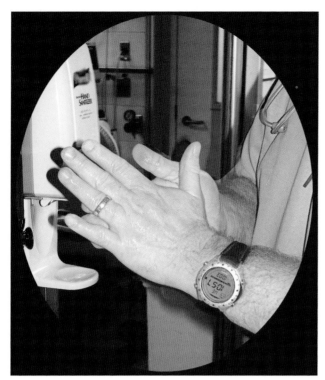

Figure 4-1. Hand washing between patient contacts.

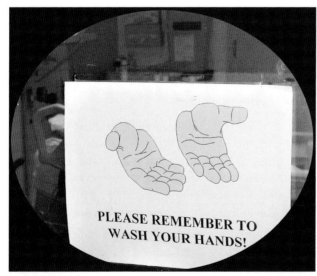

Figure 4-2. Hand hygiene reminder consistent with institutional emphasis.

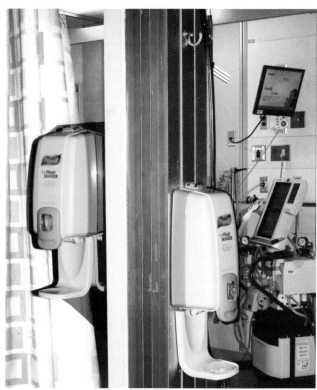

Figure 4-3. Hand antiseptic dispensers should be readily available in all patient contact areas.

—Change gloves when moving from one patient to another.

▪Recommendations for healthcare institutions

—Make improved hand hygiene adherence an institutional priority (Figure 4-2).

—Solicit multidisciplinary input in the development of policies pertaining to hand hygiene and product selection.

—Ensure ready access to alcohol-based hand rub (Figure 4-3).

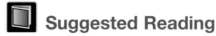 **Suggested Reading**

Guideline for hand hygiene in health care settings. *MMWR Morb Mortal Wkly Rep.* October 25, 2002;51:1–44.

CHAPTER 5

Prepping and Draping in the ICU

 ## Introduction

Preprocedural prepping and draping is essential to sterile performance of a procedure and prevention of device contamination. Proper preparation has been shown to prevent nosocomial infections and has become the subject of consensus recommendations, governmental guidelines, and regulatory review.

 ## Definitions and Terms

Skin preparation and site draping prior to performance of a procedure is intended to minimize the likelihood of either a surgical site or nosocomial infection. The goals of skin preparation are to remove soil and transient microorganisms from the skin, reduce microbial counts to subpathogenic levels in a short period of time with minimal tissue irritation, and inhibit rapid regrowth of microorganisms. Consensus guidelines have been developed by the Centre for Disease Control and Prevention (CDC) for skin and site preparation for central venous catheters which can reasonably be extrapolated to central venous devices (ie, intravascular pacing wires), central intra-arterial catheters and devices (ie, intra-aortic balloon pump). Devices at lower risk of infection (ie, peripheral intravenous catheter) can be inserted with less stringent techniques.

- Hand hygiene: See Chapter 4.

- No-touch procedure: Performance of a procedure during which the sterile portion of a device is not touched (ie, catheter portion of peripheral intravenous catheter).

- Aseptic technique: Includes the use of sterile or non-sterile gloves and a no-touch technique (ie, no contact with the portion of the device that will be inserted).

- Skin antisepsis: Depending on site, may include hair removal and skin cleansing with an antibacterial agent including povidone-iodine, chlorhexidine, or alcohol.

- Draping: A method by which the sterile area in which a procedure is to be performed is isolated from a potentially contaminated area. Options include paper, cloth, and plastic drapes. Drapes may also be used to lay out equipment used for performance of procedure.

- Maximal sterile barrier precautions: Includes cap, mask, sterile gown, sterile gloves, and large sterile drape.

 ## Techniques

- Nonsterile gloves should be worn to protect healthcare workers during the performance of any procedure in which there is a risk of contact with patient's blood, fluids, or secretions, and which does not require prep and drape (ie, nasogastric tube placement).

- Hand hygiene should be performed prior to and between all procedures as described in Chapter 4.

- Procedures that do not violate patient's defense mechanisms or wherein sterilization is infeasible (ie, cardioversion, endotracheal intubation, feeding tube placement) can be performed without prepping or draping.

- Procedures associated with minimal risk of nosocomial infection (ie, peripheral intravenous catheter placement) may be performed following skin antiseptic preparation using a no-touch procedure and without draping.

- Procedures in which the skin is violated and that are associated with high risk of nosocomial infections should be performed with maximal sterile barrier precautions including site preparation and draping.

- The operator should prepare for a procedure depending on the degree of risk to self and patient according to the following general rules:

  —Procedures with significant risk to operator (ie, from patient blood or secretions)

  • Gloves to protect hands from contact-related organisms.

- Mask to protect operator from airborne organisms (ie, high efficiency particulate air (HEPA) purifying mask with tuberculosis patient).
- Glasses to protect operator from droplet contamination to the eyes.

—Procedures with limited risk to patient (ie, skin electrode placement)

- Nonsterile gloves at operator's discretion

—Procedures with moderate risk to patient and operator (ie, peripheral venous and arterial catheter, enteral tube placement, bronchoscopy)

- Nonsterile gloves and no-touch procedure

—Procedures with significant risk to patient (ie, central venous and arterial line, ventriculostomy)

- Mask, gown, and sterile gloves

- Site should be inspected for moles, warts, and rashes which should be left undisturbed during site preparation.

- Where possible, hair should be left intact at the procedure site—inappropriate hair removal traumatizes the site and provides the opportunity for bacterial colonization.

- Hair removal can be performed with a depilatory, razor, or electric shaver; however, razors can abrade skin, depilatories can irritate skin, and an electric shaver is preferred where available.

- Soil and debris should be removed from the area around procedure site prior to application of antiseptic agents.

- Antiseptic agents should be applied using sterile supplies (ie, swabs, sponges) starting at the center of incision/insertion site and moving circularly outward to the periphery of the site to be sterilized (Figure 5-1).

- The prepared area of skin delineated by the drape should be sufficiently large to accommodate the procedure site, potential alternative sites (ie, additional

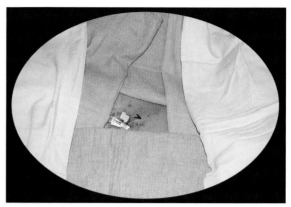

Figure 5-2. Site prepped and widely draped to permit performance of procedure without contamination of operators hands or equipment.

interspaces during performance of a lumbar puncture), and dressings.

- Sterile drapes should be applied over an area large enough to accommodate the procedure site (as described above) as well as cover a sufficient area to allow the operator to perform the procedure with no risk of equipment contamination (ie, during performance of a procedure with a long device like a pulmonary arterial catheter) (Figure 5-2).

- Sterile drapes should ideally be secured in such a way that they exclude nonsterile skin or hair from the procedure site and will not move during the performance of the procedure (ie, with an adhesive border on the underside of a fenestrated drape).

 ## Clinical Pearls and Pitfalls

- It is often challenging to perform a procedure in a critical care room due to cramped quarters and the presence of bedside devices, but it is well worth the additional time to move equipment, position the bed height, and lay out equipment so as to optimize operator comfort—a comfortable operator is more likely to be successful and efficient and less likely to make mistakes or contaminate devices.

- It is advisable to get help from an additional provider who may both monitor the patient and obtain additional equipment, if needed, so that the operator need not break sterile technique.

 ## Suggested Reading

AORN Perioperative Standards and Recommended Practices, 2008 Edition: pp 565–73.

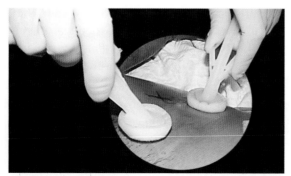

Figure 5-1. Procedure site marked and undergoing circumferential prep with antiseptic swabs.

CHAPTER 6

Informed Consent and Procedure Documentation

 Introduction

Many invasive procedures, such as central venous access and endotracheal intubation, clearly require prospective informed consent from the patient or a proxy. Other procedures may not require consent, such as enteral tube placement or urinary catheterization, although these procedures are not entirely risk-free. In practice in the ICU, it is often necessary to get consent from a proxy, because the critically ill patient is unable to give informed consent. In addition to documentation of informed consent, most procedures should be documented in the medical record and in many cases this includes the need for an insertion and a removal note.

 Definitions and Terms

- Informed consent: The legal and ethical obligation to provide a patient with information necessary to make a fully informed decision about a procedure or treatment.
- Informed consent elements:
  —Discussion of the nature of the procedure with the patient
  —Discussion of reasonable alternatives to the procedure
  —Relevant risks, benefits
  —Patient acceptance/agreement
- Implied consent: The concept that a reasonable person would choose to undergo treatment or procedure when in similar circumstances—may be applied under emergency circumstances when the patient is unable to consent and a proxy cannot be reached.
- Consent form: The document used to record the consent process, typically detailing the elements of consent as well as the signatures of the parties to the consent.

- Universal consent form: A form developed to allow the patient to consent to a number of common ICU procedures (ie, line placement, line changes, endotracheal intubation) on admission to the ICU eliminating the need for consent on a procedure-by-procedure basis (Figure 6-1).
- Healthcare proxy: An agent appointed by a patient to make medical decisions in the event that the patient is incapacitated and unable to make decisions on their own—in certain states (ie, New York), family members do not have the authority to make medical decisions for incapacitated adults.

 Techniques

- Prior to a planned procedure, the provider credentialed to perform that procedure should obtain consent from the patient or proxy, and document same in the medical record
- After the performance of the procedure, a "procedure note" should be placed in the medical record (Figure 6-2)—this note serves as a record of the time, technique, medications used, location, and complications (if any) of the procedure.
- In many cases, it is appropriate to document discontinuation of a device (ie, extubation note, discontinuation of central line) both to delimit the period of the device's use and to document the process of discontinuation and any associated problems (ie, patient self-extubation).

 Suggested Reading

Davis BS, Pohlman A, Gehlbach B, et al. Improving the process of informed consent in the critically ill. *JAMA*. 2003;289:1963–1968.

Office of the General Counsel. Informed Consent. AMA. http://www.ama-assn.org/ama/pub/category/4608.html. (Accessed on May 11, 2008.)

There may be other ways to evaluate your airway and lungs instead of performing a bronchoscopy. These include possible x-ray examinations or CT and MRI scans. However, none of these alternatives provide direct visualization of your airways and lungs or provide an opportunity for a biopsy, if needed.

If you are unsure about having an A-line, CVC or PAC inserted or about undergoing intubation or a bronchoscopy, please discuss these possible alternatives with your physician.

Agreement: The information on this from was explained to me by _____ . I understand the information and I have had the opportunity to ask any questions that I might have regarding A-line insertion, CVC insertion PAC insertion, incubation, and bronchoscopy, the reasons any of these procedures may be performed; the associated potential risks and complications to each of these procedures; and the possible alternatives. I agree to undergo any of these procedures, if needed, to be performed by _____ and his/her associates, assistants and appropriate hospital personnel and accept the risks. I also agree that fellows, residents and surgical assistants may participate in significant tasks that are part of these procedures. In addition, I agree to have any other appropriate personnel present for any of these procedures.

Signature: _____ Date: _____
            Patient

Signature: _____ Date: _____
            Physician obtaining and witnessing patient's signature

To be used if the patient is a minor, unconscious otherwise lacking decision making capacity.

I, _____ , the _____
            Name   Relationship to patient

of _____ , hereby give consent on his/her behalf.
            Patient name

Signature: _____ Date: _____
            Relative, surrogate or guardian

Signature: _____ Date: _____
            Physician

Signature: _____ Date: _____
            Witness to telephone consent

Figure 6-1. Signature portion of a universal consent for a variety of intensive care procedures.

PROCEDURE NOTE

☐ Trauna surgery service ☐ Surgical critical care ☐ Cardiothoracic critical care ☐ Neuro critical care
☐ Medical intensive care ☐ Cardiology critical care ☐ Other

Date _____ Time _____

Patient location/unit _____

Patient Identification (need 2):	Procedure Verification:	Site Marked (operative site):	Time-out with all member of procedure team immediately prior to procedure:
☐ Name/DOB ☐ Verbal with patient and/or family ☐ Other (MRN)-use when there are 2 patients with same name and DOB	☐ Procedure confirmed with patient or family/designee ☐ Consent for procedure signed ☐ Relevant documentation completed, reviewed and signed ☐ Clinical indications for procedure	☐ Yes ☐ N/A	☐ Correct patient identified ☐ Agreement on procedure ☐ Correct side and site ☐ Correct patient position ☐ Availability of correct implant/equipment or special requirements

Completed by: Name (print) _____ Signature _____

Title _____ Date _____ Time _____

Indications for procedure:

☐ Airway maintenance ☐ Hemothorax/pleural effusion ☐ Respiratory failure
☐ Arrhythrria/dysrhythmia ☐ Hyperalinentation ☐ Suspected pneumonia
☐ Cardiopulmonary arrest ☐ Laceration ☐ Venous access
☐ Enteral nutrition ☐ Lobar collapse ☐ Other _____
☐ Hermodynamic monitoring ☐ Pneumothorax

Procedure:* see additional documentation   **Critical Elements:**

☐ Bronchoscopy *   ☐ Insertion of scope, viewing, removal of scope
☐ Cardioversion   ☐ Identification of cardiac rhythm, cardioversion
☐ Central line insertion (large bore)*   ☐ Venipuncture, catheter insertion
☐ Central line insertion (triple lumen)*   ☐ Venipuncture, catheter insertion
☐ Chest tube insertion   ☐ Skin incision, plenral entry, tube placement
☐ CPR*   ☐ Assessing patient, establishing airway, restoring breathing and circulation defibrillation
☐ Endotracbeal incubation   ☐ Insertion of laryngoscope, placement of endotracheal tube, removal of laryngoscope
☐ Insertion of enteral feeding tube with fluoroscopic guidance   ☐ Insertion of tube, positioning of tube with fluorosopic guidance
☐ Laceration repair   ☐ Wound assessment, preparation, and repair
    Length _____ ☐ Simple ☐ Complex   ☐ Incision, insertion of dilators, insertion of tracheostomy tube
☐ Percutaneous tracheostomy*   ☐ Insertion or pulmonary artery catheter, measurement of cardiac output and/or PA pressure
☐ Pulmonary arterial catheter
☐ Other _____   ☐ Other _____

Description/comment (catheter type, location, each vein (attempted) commulated, suture type, device size, x-ray confirmation of catheter, reason for catheter removed) _____

_____

_____

☐ Anesthesia (local) _____ ☐ (IV-conscious sedation) _____
Sequence _____ Sample sent _____

I personally supervised Dr. _____ (resident/fellow) in the performance of the documented procedure. I was present for the critical element of this procedure and was immediately available for the entire procedure.

_____   _____
     Attending physician signature   Printed name/beeper number

DO NOT USE UNAPPROVED ABBREVIATION

Figure 6-2. Intensive care procedure documentation template.

CHAPTER 7

Critical Care Transport

 ## Introduction

Intensive care unit (ICU) patients are at their most vulnerable during the period of transport to and from the ICU.

 ## Definitions and Terms

- Transport: Includes travel to the unit from the floor, emergency room, or operating room and from the unit to the floor, operating room, and off-site test and procedure locations.

 ## Techniques

- Prior to transport, the transferring personnel should ensure that the receiving personnel has received report on the patient's status, if applicable.

- If the patient is going off-site for a test or procedure, the stability of the patient should be evaluated immediately prior to transport to ensure that the requirement for the test outweighs the risk inherent in the transport.

- Prior to transport, all relevant data should be reviewed to ensure that the performance of a planned procedure will not put the patient at additional risk (ie, does the patient have an intravenous [IV] contrast allergy).

- Where applicable, lower risk alternatives that can be performed in the ICU should be considered (ie, portable anterior-posterior chest x-ray in ICU vs. formal posterior-anterior and lateral in radiology department).

- Are adequate numbers of skilled personnel available to make the trip safely and is adequate coverage available in the ICU?

- Appropriate medications and an administration route (ie, patent IV line) should be identified prior to transport.
  - Make sure resuscitation medications are available where appropriate (ie, atropine).

  - Make sure all infusion medications are sufficiently full to last through planned transport or that replacement supplies are available.

- Additional equipment needed for safe transport should be available (ie, portable suction for chest tubes).

- Nursing interventions should be performed prior to transport to diminish the risk of nosocomial infections.
  - Keep head of bed elevated during transport where possible to diminish the risk of regurgitation and aspiration.
  - Empty urinary drainage bag to prevent reflux of urine into the bladder.

- Evaluate ventilatory status prior to transport to ensure that ICU ventilatory and oxygen support can be reproduced both during transport and at receiving site.

- Are adequate oxygen supplies available during transport (check cylinder supply)?

- Is a portable ventilator necessary to reproduce positive end-expiratory pressure (PEEP) or ventilator mode during transport?

- Is there a ventilator at destination?

- Is there a face mask with a self-reinflating resuscitation bag immediately available?

 ## Clinical Pearls and Pitfalls

- A checklist (Figure 7-1), analogous to those used on commercial aircraft prior to take-off and landings, can be used to ensure that all elements are in place to transport a patient safely.

- The transition from mechanical to manual ventilation can be problematic under the following circumstances:
  - Derecruitment of the lung and consequent problems with oxygenation.
  - Manual overventilation, with consequent air trapping or auto-PEEP and decreased venous return

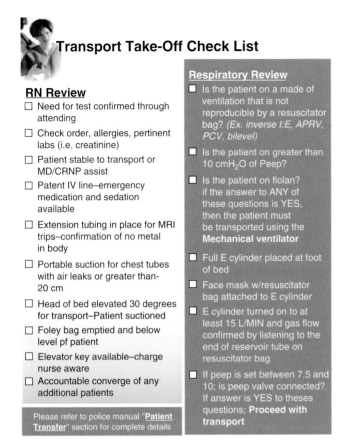

Transport Take-Off Check List

RN Review

- ☐ Need for test confirmed through attending
- ☐ Check order, allergies, pertinent labs (i.e. creatinine)
- ☐ Patient stable to transport or MD/CRNP assist
- ☐ Patent IV line–emergency medication and sedation available
- ☐ Extension tubing in place for MRI trips–confirmation of no metal in body
- ☐ Portable suction for chest tubes with air leaks or greater than-20 cm
- ☐ Head of bed elevated 30 degrees for transport–Patient suctioned
- ☐ Foley bag emptied and below level pf patient
- ☐ Elevator key available–charge nurse aware
- ☐ Accountable converge of any additional patients

Please refer to police manual "**Patient Transfer**" section for complete details

Respiratory Review

- ☐ Is the patient on a made of ventilation that is not reproducible by a resuscitator bag? *(Ex. inverse I:E, APRV, PCV, bilevel)*
- ☐ Is the patient on greater than 10 cmH$_2$O of Peep?
- ☐ Is the patient on flolan? if the answer to ANY of these questions is YES, then the patient must be transported using the **Mechanical ventilator**
- ☐ Full E cylinder placed at foot of bed
- ☐ Face mask w/resuscitator bag attached to E cylinder
- ☐ E cylinder turned on to at least 15 L/MIN and gas flow confirmed by listening to the end of reservoir tube on resuscitator bag
- ☐ If peep is set between 7.5 and 10; is peep valve connected? If answer is YES to theses questions; **Proceed with transport**

Figure 7-1. Intensive care transportation checklist. *Copyright Trustees of the University of Pennsylvania, with permission.*

leading to hypotension—this is readily diagnosed by disconnecting the ventilator and allowing trapped air to be exhaled, which will result in prompt improvement in blood pressure.

Suggested Reading

Lahner D, Nikolic A, Marhofer P, et al. Incidence of complications in intrahospital transport of critically ill patients—experience in an Austrian university. *Wien Kilin Wochenschr.* 2007;119:412–416.

CHAPTER 8

Cardiopulmonary Resuscitation

 Introduction

Cardiopulmonary resuscitation (CPR) is a common therapy in the intensive care unit (ICU), and begins with standard advanced cardiac life support (ACLS) algorithms as published by American Heart Association guidelines, which were designed for application in non-ICU settings, often proceeding to more advanced therapies.

 Definitions and Terms

- Respiratory arrest: Cessation of effective breathing due to a variety of causes including airway obstruction, drugs, central nervous system pathology, or intrinsic pulmonary disease
- Cardiac arrest: Cessation of effective circulation due to a variety of causes including arrhythmias, primary cardiac muscle failure, pericardial disease, thoracic pathology (ie, pneumo- or hemothorax), and circulatory incompetence (ie, hemorrhage, sepsis, anaphylaxis)
- Airway: The establishment of a patent airway
- Breathing: Encompasses both ventilation and oxygenation
- Circulation: Encompasses both cardiac and vascular function

 Techniques

- The indications for CPR in an ICU are identical to those in any other setting, that is, loss of airway, breathing, and/or circulation.
- As with resuscitation in any patient, advanced directive should be evaluated prior to initiation of resuscitation to ascertain whether there are any limitations to such as "Do not intubate" or "No cardiopulmonary resuscitation."

- In many cases, the need for intervention will be identified by an alarm from one of the bedside physiologic monitors unless cardiac or respiratory arrest is witnessed.
  —Respiratory arrest—typically identified by pulse oximeter alarm, bradycardia, or respiratory rate alarm.
  —Cardiac arrest or arrhythmia—identified by automated arrhythmia detection or blood pressure alarm.
- In the event of respiratory arrest, the patient should be assessed for the presence or absence of spontaneous respiratory efforts and airway patency.
  —A patent airway should be established using maneuvers such as head and neck positioning, oral or nasal airways, and endotracheal intubation if appropriate.
  —Ventilation should be established with a resuscitation bag and/or mechanical ventilator if appropriate.
- In the event of cardiac arrest, the patient should be assessed for the presence or absence of an effective electrical rhythm.
  —In the event that there is a rhythm, the patient should be assessed for a pulse either by palpation, manometry, or arterial line tracing.
  —If there is an effective rhythm, but no pulse, the typical causes for electromechanical dissociation should be assessed including tension pneumothorax, pericardial tamponade, and hypovolemia.
  —In the event that an effective rhythm is absent, initial resuscitations should be directed toward the resumption of circulation using chest compressions (Figure 8-1), pacing, defibrillation (Figure 8-2), and/or cardioversion as warranted.
- Blood tests should be secured as soon as feasible to evaluate oxygenation; ventilation; acid-base status; serum hemoglobin; and electrolytes, including potassium, magnesium, and calcium.

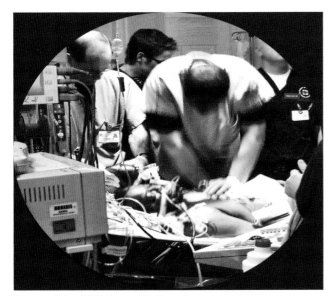

Figure 8-1. CPR in an ICU patient.

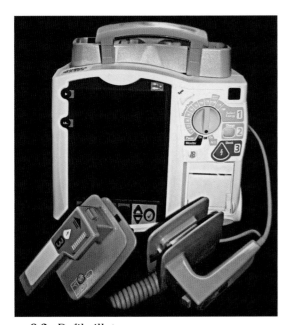

Figure 8-2. Defibrillator.

■ Resuscitation should proceed in accordance with ACLS algorithms to the extent they are applicable in specific ICU patients.

 Clinical Pearls and Pitfalls

■ Unlike many regular patient floor rooms, ICU rooms are typically equipped with resuscitation bags, suction, oxygen delivery systems. The time between recognition of a cardiopulmonary arrest and intervention is usually brief, enhancing the likelihood of successful resuscitation.

■ Certain standard ACLS interventions may be inappropriate in certain ICU populations:

—Chest compressions may be contraindicated after certain cardiac surgical procedures, that is, valve replacement, in which compressions may cause tearing of suture lines—in this case open cardiac massage is the preferred intervention.

—Direct laryngoscopy may be relatively contraindicated in certain patient populations, that is, laryngeal or tracheal surgery, where bronchoscopically directed airway management preferred.

■ The effectiveness of chest compressions can be monitored on arterial line tracings when available.

■ Excessive manual ventilation can cause auto-PEEP and insufficient venous return to the heart.

■ Correct endotracheal tube position should be confirmed with carbon dioxide detection devices, although these devices may be inaccurate in full circulatory arrest and the absence of effective circulation.

■ Potential pharmacologic causes, (ie, narcotics, potassium overdose, wrong, or runaway infusion) for cardiopulmonary arrest should be considered early in any ICU patient because of the higher than normal likelihood of exposure to pharmacologic interventions in this population.

 Suggested Reading

2005 American Heart Association Guidelines for Cardiopulmonary Resuscitation and Emergency Cardiovascular Care. *Circulation*. 2005;112:1–203. www.americanheart.org/eccguidelines. (Accessed on May 11, 2008.)

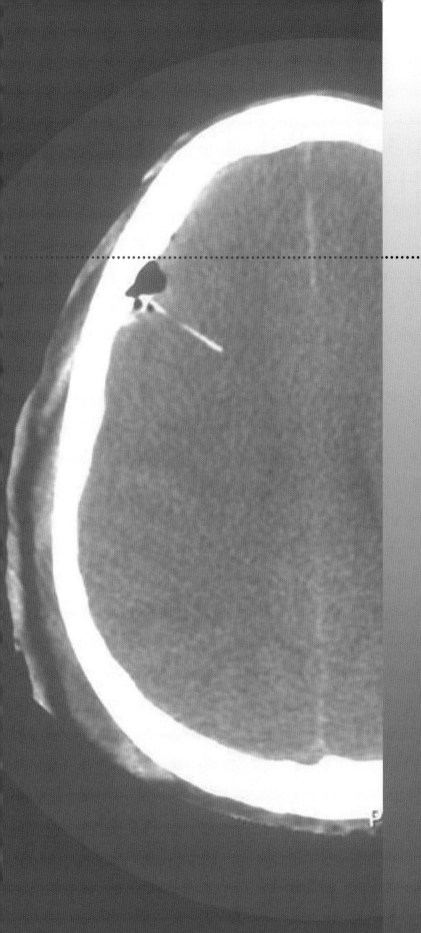

Neurological Procedures

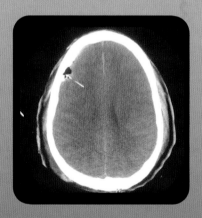

CHAPTER 9

Pain Management in the ICU

Introduction

Intensive care patients experience pain to varying degrees and for a variety of reasons during their intensive care unit (ICU) stay. The evolution of the discipline of pain management as well as increasingly precise knowledge about the pharmacology and physiology of pain has led to significant advances in its evaluation and treatment. Intensive care providers have a growing arsenal of tools with which to treat pain including pain management consultants, patient-controlled analgesia (PCA), epidural analgesia, opioids, and new nonsteroidal agents.

Definitions and Terms

- Pain: The sensation of discomfort or distress, which may be localized or diffuse, resulting from stimulation of pain receptors (or nociceptors), and which results in the initiation of a variety of protective and potentially deleterious physiologic consequences.

- Pain scale: A variety of visual analogs, indexes, and questionnaires designed to help a patient characterize the intensity, location, and quality of pain.

- Visual analog scale: Probably the most common approach to pain assessment in intensive care patients (Figure 9-1).

- PCA: See Figure 9-2.

- PCEA: Patient-controlled epidural analgesia (Figure 9-3).

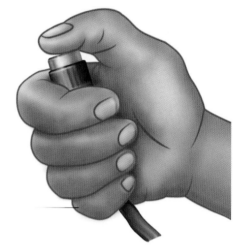

Figure 9-2. Patient-controlled device for intravenous and epidural analgesic regimens. Patients can administer a bolus of the drug on demand by pushing the button.

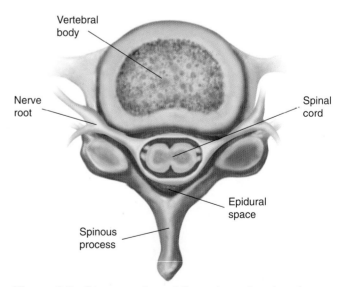

Figure 9-3. Cross-section of the spine, showing the epidural space distended with infused fluid and adjacent to nerve roots as they emerge from the cord.

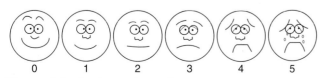

Figure 9-1. Analog pain scale.

Techniques

- Intensive care patients experience pain due to the underlying illness, injury, or therapy (ie, surgery), which may be augmented by sleeplessness or anxiety.
- Pain evaluation is a routine and required part of intensive care nursing assessment, and assessment may take the form of direct questioning, the use of scales and charts or empiric/clinical evaluation when the patient is unable to participate directly in the assessment.
- Pain may result in adverse secondary clinical consequences such as splinting (and consequent atelectasis), tachycardia, sleeplessness, and delirium that may guide the choice of the primary treatment and require the use of complementary treatments to ameliorate the secondary problem (ie, β-blockade, sleeping medication)
- Narcotic agents are typically used as first-line interventions in the ICU and can be administered intravenously by bolus, continuous infusion, patient-controlled continuous infusion, or as components of epidural analgesia
- Nonsteroidal anti-inflammatory agents can be used to supplement narcotics
- Initial assessment on admission to the intensive care should include consideration of the admission diagnosis, the likelihood that the patient will experience pain during the ICU stay, preadmission narcotic use that may necessitate modification of the analgesic regiment (ie, patient's long-term narcotics use at home), cultural factors (ie, willingness to admit pain), and the patient's ability to communicate.
- Admission orders to the ICU should include the prescription of pain medications to be administered on an as-needed basis or continuously and typically provide the bedside provider or patient with the ability to administer bolus doses prior to painful procedures or nursing interventions (ie, turning, dressing changes, etc.).

- Patient-controlled analgesic regimens (ie, PCA and PCEA) are typically prescribed with a "basal" (ie, background, continuous) infusion rate, a "demand" bolus dose (administered when patient pushes hand-held button), along with a "lockout" interval, which describes the minimal interval between effective demand boluses (so that the patient cannot administer an overdose by repeatedly pushing the button).
- Local anesthetic agents may be combined with narcotics in PCEA infusions and may act synergistically in pain relief, although either class of drug can be administered individually in a PCEA infusion.

 Clinical Pearls and Pitfalls

- Patients on chronic opioids will have higher requirements for opioids in hospital and doses should be adjusted accordingly.
- Match the therapy and drug to the anticipated duration of the need for pain management—longer acting drugs should be used for longer duration therapy.
- Preemptive treatment (ie, before pain becomes severe) may paradoxically decrease the requirement for pain medication.
- Pain management should be titrated to facilitate activities that will prevent patient complications (ie, suctioning, coughing, turning, mobilization) without causing inappropriate sedation.

 Suggested Readings

Burton AW, Eappen S. Regional anesthesia techniques for pain control in the intensive care unit. *Crit Care Clin.* 1999;15:77–88.

Liu LL, Gropper MA. Postoperative analgesia and sedation in the adult intensive care unit: a guide to drug selection. *Drugs.* 2003;63:755–767.

Mularski RA. Pain management in the intensive care unit. *Crit Care Clin.* 2004;20:381–401.

Schulz-Stubner S. The critically ill patient and regional anesthesia. *Curr Opin Anesthesiol.* 2006;19:538–544.

CHAPTER 10

Agitation Scale

 Introduction

Anxiety, pain, and delirium are common in intensive care patients and may be due any one of or combinations of the following factors: disorientation, medications, or the underlying disease. While anxiety can often be relieved by compassionate staff, agitation and delirium can result in patient actions that put them at risk for falls, dislodgement of medical devices, or disruption of wound dressings and incisions. Appropriate management of these problems requires early identification, differentiation among the potential causes, and appropriate treatment.

 Definitions and Terms

- Anxiety: An unpleasant emotional state consisting of a set of mental and physiologic responses to anticipated real or imagined danger—the mental responses include apprehension, tension while the physiologic responses include increased heart rate, respiratory rate, sweating, weakness, and fatigue.
- Delirium: An acute, short-term disturbance in consciousness characterized by disorganized thoughts, inability to focus attention, disorientation, sensory misperceptions and may result in paranoid ideation, sleep disturbances, excessive or inappropriate motor activity, and memory impairment.
- Agitation: Excessive, purposeless cognition and movement manifested as restlessness.
- Agitation scale: One of several scales designed to provide caregivers with a uniform, objective measure of a patient's mental status—common scales in use include:
  —Ramsey scale
    Ranges from no response at one extreme to agitated and restless at the other (six-point scale: 1–6)
  —Riker sedation agitation scale
    Ranges from unarousable to dangerous agitation (seven-point scale: 1–7)
  —Motor activity assessment scale

    Ranges from unresponsive to dangerously agitated (seven-point scale: 0–6)
  —Richmond agitation sedation scale
    Ranges from sedated to combative at the other and includes verbal and physical stimuli (ten-point scale: –5 to 4)

 Techniques

- Agitation scales are typically applied at the bedside by medical providers.
- Treatment for agitation, disorientation, and delirium typically requires treatment of the underlying problem where identifiable.
- Anxiety and disorientation can be treated with reassurance, reorientation, recreation of a familiar environment with props such as pictures, assistance from family members, friends, and others.
- Anxiolytics such as benzodiazepines can be used when nonpharmacologic alternatives are insufficient or inadequate.
- Benzodiazepines are often useful in the management of drug or alcohol withdrawal.
- Antipsychotic agents such as haloperidol can be used in patients with delirium refractory to other interventions.
- Pain and sleep medications should be used when pain or sleeplessness are possible contributors.

 Clinical Pearls and Pitfalls

- Critically ill patients may be "disoriented" for a variety of reasons including:
  —Neurological process such as head injury, encephalitis, and so on.
  —Drug side effect.
  —Dementia, which may be subclinical in a patient's home environment but become manifest during a hospitalization—this typically occurs in the elderly.

—Drug or alcohol intoxication.

—Drug or alcohol withdrawal.

▪ The differential diagnosis for delirium includes many of same processes causing disorientation as well as:

—Focal seizures

—Primary psychiatric processes such as depression, mania

—Sleep deprivation

—Systemic and intracranial infection/sepsis

—Fever

—Electrolyte and metabolic disturbances

▪ Delirium is characterized by inattention—a patient who is able to focus attention on the examiner is not delirious.

▪ Untreated delirium is associated with an increased incidence of both ICU and hospital comorbidities and death.

▪ Some recent data suggest that delirium experienced during an intensive care admission may have significant long-term consequences and be associated with an increased incidence of posthospitalization dementia.

▪ Wrist (Figure 10-1), ankle (Figure 10-2), and torso restraints may sometimes be necessary in the initial management of agitation and delirium, both for provider and patient safety—the indication for restraints should be documented in a medical order and the requirement reevaluated on a regular basis as per regional regulatory requirements.

▪ Agitated patients are at high risk for falls and accidental decannulation (ie, lines, tubes, etc.) and typically require extra vigilance and close monitoring to prevent same.

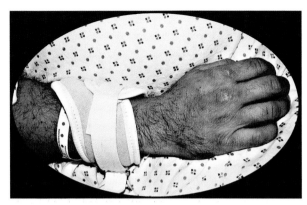

Figure 10-1. Padded wrist restraint.

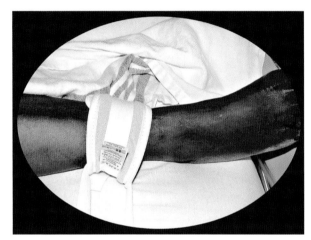

Figure 10-2. Padded ankle restraint.

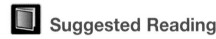 **Suggested Reading**

Pun BT, Ely EW. The importance of diagnosing and managing ICU delirium. *Chest.* 2007;132:624–636.

CHAPTER 11

Glasgow Coma Score

Introduction

The Glasgow Coma Score (or GCS) is a neurological scale used in many settings to objectively classify the level of consciousness of patients. It was initially developed for head-injured patients, but its use has been extrapolated to chronically critically ill patients, and it is one component of several different intensive care severity scoring systems (Figure 11-1).

Definitions and Terms

- Eye response: Eye opening in response to various levels of stimulus
- Verbal response: Verbal communication in terms of comprehensibility
- Motor response: Movement in response to various stimuli

Techniques

- Eye response (E)
  - No eye opening = 1
  - Eye opening in response to pain (ie, pressure on fingernail bed, mandible, supraorbital area, or sternum) = 2
  - Eye opening to speech = 3
  - Spontaneous eye opening = 4
- Verbal response (V)
  - No verbal response = 1
  - Incomprehensible sounds (ie, moaning) = 2
  - Inappropriate words (ie, random sounds or speech) = 3
  - Confused, coherent speech (ie, disorientation or confusion) = 4
  - Oriented = 5
- Motor (M)
  - No movements = 1
  - Extension in response to painful stimuli (ie, decerebrate posturing) = 2
  - Flexion in response to pain (ie, decorticate posturing) = 3
  - Flexion withdrawal in response to pain (ie, withdrawal of body part in response to stimulus) = 4
  - Localized movements in response to pain (ie, purposeful movements across midline toward painful stimulus) = 5
  - Obeys commands = 6
- GCS less than or equal to 8 is consistent with severe brain injury when applied to head injured population.
- GCS 9 to 12 consistent with moderate brain injury.
- GCS greater than or equal to 13 consistent with minor injury.
- Modifiers are used in the presence of severe eye/facial swelling, spinal cord injury, or oral intubation to indicate that that portion of the exam cannot be performed (ie, 11T indicates a normal eye and motor exam in an intubated patient).

Category		Score
Eye opening	Spontaneous	4
	To speech	3
	To pain	2
	None	1
Verbal response	Oriented	5
	Confused	4
	Inappropriate	3
	Incomprehensible	2
	None	1
Motor response	Obeys commands	6
	Localizes	5
	Withdraws	4
	Flexion/decorticate	3
	Extension/decrebrate	2
	None	1
Total score		15

Figure 11-1. The Glasgow coma scale.

Clinical Pearls and Pitfalls

- Some examiners break the score down by individual components (ie, E4V5M6) to precisely specify the components of the exam.

- A variety of independent factors may interfere with the applicability of the GCS to traumatic brain injury because they act as confounders, such as intoxication, sepsis, and shock.

- Alternative scores have been developed for use in children of various ages.

- The GCS has been used successfully to predict outcome in a variety of settings

Suggested Reading

Wijdicks EF. Clinical scales for comatose patients: the Glasgow Coma Scale in historical context and the new FOUR score. *Rev Neurol Dis.* 2006;3:109–117.

CHAPTER 12

Neuromuscular Blockade

 ## Introduction

Therapeutic neuromuscular blockade is a routine part of intraoperative anesthetic management for many surgeries and is occasionally appropriate in the ICU in order to facilitate certain forms of mechanical ventilation, prevent patient movements that may harm the patient, facilitate procedures, decrease oxygen consumption, or prevent muscle spasm in certain diseases. Therapeutic paralysis involves the administration of neuromuscular blocking agents to interfere with the synaptic transmission at the neuromuscular junction and thereby prevent or decrease the force of muscle contractions. These drugs are administered in boluses or by continuous infusion and their effects can be monitored by patient observation or with peripheral nerve stimulators similar to those used in the operating room.

 ## Definitions and Terms

- Neuromuscular blocking agent: A drug that interferes with normal acetylcholine-mediated synaptic transmission (Figure 12-1) by blocking acetylcholine's actions at the postsynaptic receptors (Figure 12-2).

- Depolarizing neuromuscular blocking agents (ie, succinylcholine) depolarize the neuromuscular junction causing initial release of acetylcholine followed by paralysis, and are *not* typically used in the ICU because of their very short duration and the potential for potassium release on administration.

- Non–depolarizing muscle-blocking agents (NMBs) interfere with the action of acetylcholine at the postsynaptic receptor and *are* typically used for ICU administration.

- Train-of-four (TOF) monitoring is a technique by which the effects of NMBs can be monitored objectively involving the administration of a series of four successive electrical stimulations over a peripheral nerve. The force of contraction of a muscle enervated by that nerve is monitored (Figure 12-3) and monitoring can be performed at a variety of locations (Figure 12-4).

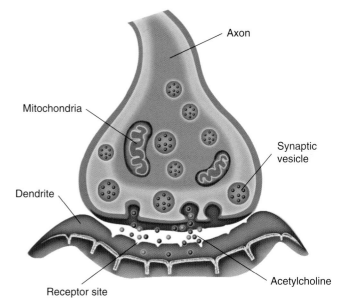

Figure 12-1. Normal synaptic transmission, where acetylcholine (orange circles) acts as the neurotransmitter from the nerve to the muscle.

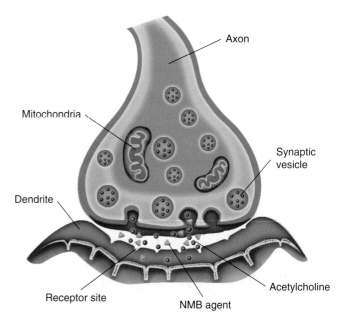

Figure 12-2. Paralytic agents (green triangles) interfere with the actions of acetylcholine in the junction.

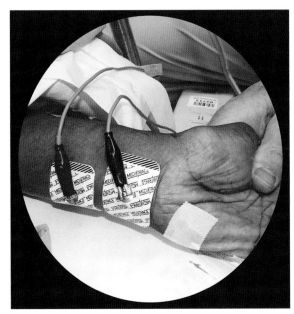

Figure 12-3. The degree of paralysis is monitored by administering a series of electrical impulses over a nerve and monitoring the contraction of a muscle enervated by that nerve (ulnar nerve and thumb contraction in this case).

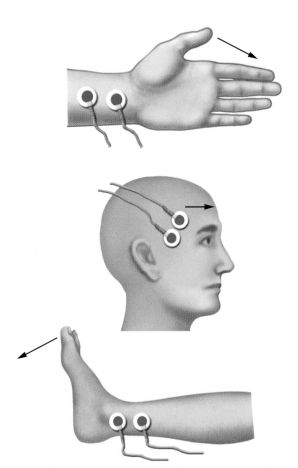

Figure 12-4. Several common sites for monitoring in the ICU including the wrist, the forehead, and the ankle.

 Techniques

- Clinical indications

  —Chemical paralysis is indicated to facilitate certain nonphysiologic approaches to mechanical ventilation such as inverse-ratio ventilation, airway pressure-release ventilation, or independent lung-ventilation that may be indicated in diseases such as adult respiratory distress syndrome (ARDS) or obstructive pulmonary diseases.

  —Paralysis may be indicated to prevent the patient from muscle movements that may result in harmful consequences, such as evisceration in a patient with an open abdomen or neck movement following a tracheal anastomosis.

  —Paralysis is indicated for the performance of procedures in the ICU such as endotracheal intubation.

  —Short-term paralysis may be indicated for optimal performance of diagnostic procedures such as radiographic imaging.

  —Paralysis may be indicated to decrease oxygen consumption in patients with precarious oxygen delivery and shivering.

  —Paralysis is indicated in certain unusual diseases such as tetanus and neuroleptic malignant syndrome.

- Therapeutic paralysis

  —Determine indication for paralysis.

  —Ensure that patient has an artificial airway and is on a ventilator mode that will ensure adequate ventilation following administration of paralytic and consequent cessation of spontaneous ventilation and triggering of ventilator.

  —Ensure that patient is receiving both adequate sedation (ie, benzodiazepine) and analgesia (ie, narcotic) prior to initiation of paralytic therapy.

  —Initiate treatment with NMB paralytic: The agent is typically chosen based on institutional protocols and organ dysfunctions that may affect elimination half-life (ie, pancuronium and renal failure).

  —NMBs may be administered by intermittent bolus, bolus followed by infusion, or by infusion (without bolus).

  —NMBs are typically titrated to one twitch in four (Figure 12-5).

  —NMBs are typically stopped briefly every 24 to 48 hours to reassess the need for paralytic therapy.

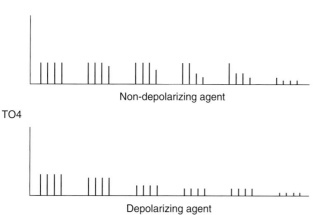

Figure 12-5. The onset of paralysis over time, showing muscle contraction amplitude in response to sets of four electrical stimuli by a twitch monitor comparing non–depolarizing agents (ie, pancuronium) with depolarizing agents (ie, succinylcholine).

 ## Clinical Pearls and Pitfalls

- A small percentage of patients treated with paralytics in the ICU have been shown to develop long-lasting weakness that has been shown to be due to several mechanisms, including delayed clearance, myopathy, or polyneuropathy.
- Prolonged clearance of NMBs in critically ill patients is typically due to organ failure in the organs responsible for elimination of the administered paralytic agent
- Myopathy following paralysis with NMB is characterized by weakness with preserved sensation, and has characteristic findings on electromyography.
- Concomitant administration of corticosteroids or aminoglycoside antibiotics has been shown to be associated with myopathy following NMB administration.
- Critical care polyneuropathy also has distinct findings on electromyography and may occur in the absence of NMB administration.
- TOF monitoring requires training and it is important to select appropriate nerve/muscle pairs for evaluation: (Figure 12-4)
  —Ulnar nerve and adductor pollicis (thumb flexion)
  —Posterior tibial nerve and flexor hallucis brevis (great toe flexion)
  —Facial nerve and corrugator supercilii (pulls eyebrow down and in producing vertical wrinkles in forehead)

 ## Suggested Reading

Sardesai AM, Griffiths R. Monitoring techniques: neuromuscular blockade. *Anesthesia and Intensive Care Medicine.* 2005;6:198–200.

CHAPTER 13

Lumbar Puncture

 ## Introduction

A lumbar puncture or spinal tap is usually performed to obtain cerebrospinal fluid (CSF) and thereby diagnose various central nervous system infectious and inflammatory diseases (ie, meningitis, encephalitis, Guillain-Barré syndrome), to evaluate CSF pressure (pseudotumor cerebri), or to administer medications (ie, antibiotics, chemotherapeutic agents).

 ## Definitions and Terms

- Interspace: The space between two spinous processes of adjacent vertebral bodies, which are referred to by a letter corresponding to which portion (cervical, thoracic, and lumbar) of the spine and which number vertebral body of that portion—L4 is the fourth lumbar vertebra, and the L4-5 interspace lies between the fourth and fifth lumbar vertebral bodies as well as being the typical location for lumbar puncture (Figure 13-1).

- Spinous process: Posteriorly protruding bony portion of the vertebra, which is typically palpable through the skin of the back in the midline.

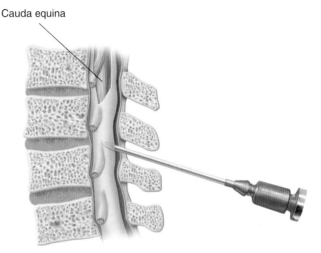

Figure 13-2. Diagram showing lumbar puncture needle entering CSF below cauda equina.

- Laminae: The two struts that join to form the spinous process and thereby form the "roof" of the spinal canal.

- Cauda equina: The lower end of the spinal cord, which typically ends between L2 and L3 (Figure 13-2).

- Dura: The leathery membrane that is the outer layer of the meninges, envelopes the brain and spinal cord and contains the CSF.

- Spinal needle: A long needle typically between 25 and 22 gauge and used to sample CSF percutaneously.

- Introducer needle: A larger needle through which a small gauge spinal needle may be passed to prevent bending during performance of the procedure.

- Obturator needle: A solid needle used to occlude the bore of the spinal needle and thereby prevent blockage with a plug of skin or tissue while the spinal needle is advanced—the obturator needle is removed to determine whether there is CSF flow through the central bore of the spinal needle.

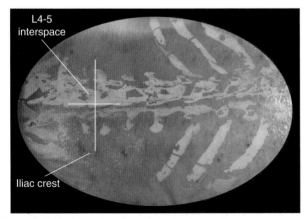

Figure 13-1. The lumbar spine in a patient in the right lateral decubitus position, showing the location of the L4-5 interspace and the posterior iliac crests.

 ## Techniques

- Consent, wash hands, prepare, and drape patient and perform universal protocol.

- Position patient for procedure: Lateral decubitus or sitting positions are both acceptable.

- Prepare and drape area around L4-5 interspace (typically at the level of the posterior superior iliac crests)—this interspace is below the distal end (cauda equina) of the spinal cord in adults and at the level of the posterior iliac crests (Figure 13-3).

- Palpate L4-5 interspace and infiltrate skin and subcutaneous tissue with local anesthetic agent.

- Insert spinal needle (directly or through introducer needle) in midline (Figures 13-4 to 13-6) aiming in a slightly cephalad direction (ie, toward the body of the L4 vertebra).

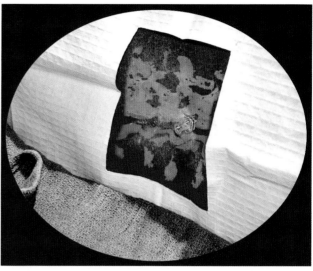

Figure 13-5. The introducer needle in place.

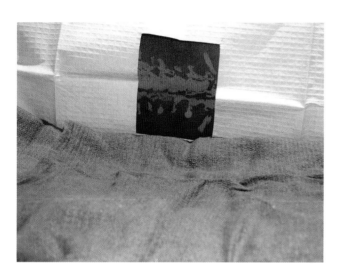

Figure 13-3. The lumbar puncture site prepped and draped.

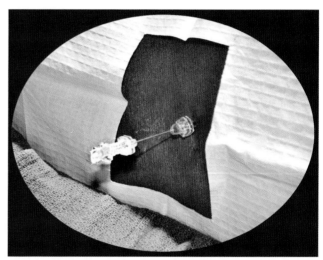

Figure 13-6. The lumbar puncture need passed through the introducer needle with a drop of CSF draining from the needle.

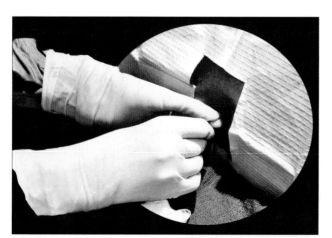

Figure 13-4. Insertion of the introducer needle (through which a smaller lumbar puncture needle can be passed).

- Advance the needle in small increments, removing the obturator needle periodically to check for CSF flow and replacing it prior to advancing—a palpable change in resistance may be felt as the needle passes through the dura (particularly with larger needles).

- The needle may need to be withdrawn and repositioned if it hits bone or causes unilateral radiating pain (paresthesia) in a nerve root distribution—suggesting that the needle tip has deviated laterally during passage and hit a nerve root.

- Once the needle passes through the dura, CSF should flow freely.

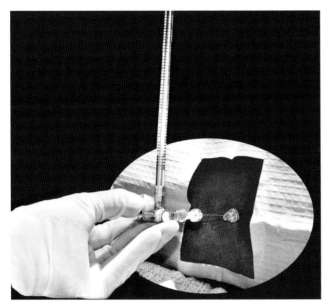

Figure 13-7. A manometer attached to the lumbar puncture needle to measure CSF pressure.

- CSF pressure should be measured (Figure 13-7) immediately (if appropriate) prior to the drainage of any quantity of CSF (Figure 13-8), so as to accurately reflect baseline CSF pressure—most lumbar puncture kits are equipped with a column manometer.
- CSF may be bloody initially if a vessel is injured during passage, but will typically clear quickly in the absence of pathology (ie, intracerebral hemorrhage).

- The desired amount of CSF should be collected in one or more containers to allow diagnostic studies (if appropriate).
- CSF drainage (pseudotumor cerebri) or medication administration (chemotherapy) may be indicated for certain diseases.
- When all desired studies are completed, the needle should be withdrawn and a small dressing can be placed over the site.

Clinical Pearls and Pitfalls

- Post-lumbar puncture, headache (spinal headache) is a relatively common complication, and due to continued drainage of CSF through the puncture site in the dura, which typically resolves with hydration and recumbency (to reduce the transdural pressure gradient).
- The use of smaller gauge and noncutting needles reduces the incidence of spinal headache.
- If a cutting needle is used, the cutting plane should be oriented with the bevel parallel to the long axis of the spine to reduce shearing of the dural fibers which run vertically.
- It may be difficult or impossible to pass the spinal needle in the midline in patients with lumbar osteophytes or compression, and the paramedian approach may be used as an alternative (Figures 13-9 and 13-10).

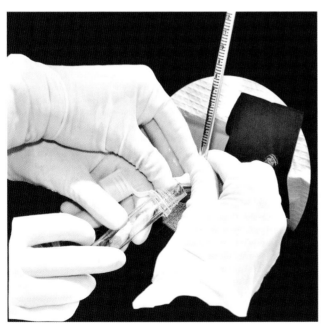

Figure 13-8. Drainage of CSF into sample vial for analysis.

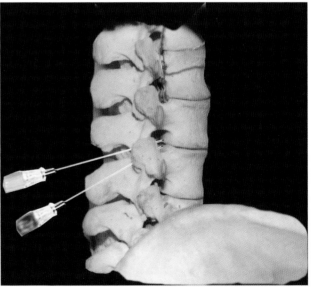

Figure 13-9. Lateral view of two approaches to lumbar puncture illustrated by the yellow (midline) needle and the red (paramedian) needle. The paramedian needle is typically passed at a slightly steeper (ie, more cephalad) angle.

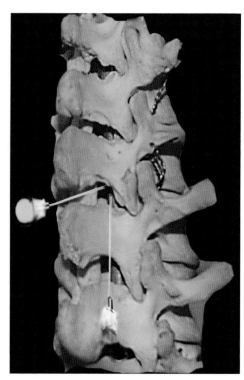

Figure 13-10. Inferoposterolateral view of the two approaches to lumbar puncture shown in Figure 13-9. The paramedian approach starts more laterally and inferiorly, and the needle is advanced over the lamina into the spinal canal.

▪ Standard medical texts should be consulted for normal CSF values and pressures and the differential diagnosis of abnormal findings.

 Suggested Reading

Greig PR, Goroszeniuk D. Role of computed tomography before lumbar puncture: a survey of clinical practice. *Postgrad Med Journal.* 2006;82:162–165.

CHAPTER 14

Brain Death Examination

Introduction

The concept that death can be diagnosed by neurologic as well as cardiac criteria has been codified by law in the United States in the Uniform Declaration of Death Act. Neurologic "brain" death is particularly relevant to intensive care unit (ICU) care, where cardiac and ventilatory function can be maintained in the absence of brain function. Brain death is the primary requirement for organ donation, although heart-beating and non–heart-beating donors contribute to the donor organ pool. In adults, the primary causes of brain death are traumatic brain injury and subarachnoid hemorrhage, whereas pediatric donors are typically abuse victims. Brain death was first defined in 1968 by an ad hoc committee at the Harvard Medical School based on clinical criteria, and has subsequently undergone redefinition by a variety of national and international bodies. While the specifics vary, the requirements have in common the requirements that the patient be in an irreversible coma, in which the cause is known, the clinical examination is consistent with brain stem death, confounding factors have been ruled out, and confirmatory tests are consistent with the foregoing.

Definitions and Terms

- Coma: A state of unconsciousness from which the patient cannot be aroused even with stimulation such as pressure on the supraorbital nerve, temporomandibular angle of the mandible, sternum, or nailbed.

- Irreversible coma: Coma wherein reversible causes such as acid-base, electrolyte, endocrine disturbances, hypothermia (core temperature < 32°C), drug intoxication, hypotension, poisoning, and pharmacological neuromuscular blockade have been ruled out as potential causes or contributors.

- Cause: Etiology of the coma.

- Brain stem examination: A series of tests in which the function and reflexes of the mesencephalon, pons, and medulla oblongata are tested.

- Confirmatory tests: Radiologic and laboratory tests used to confirm brain death, including cerebral angiography, electroencephalography, transcranial Doppler ultrasonography, cerebral scintigraphy, as well as serum drug levels.

Techniques

- Clinical tests

  —Absence of motor responses to painful stimuli.

  —Absence of light reflex on pupillary examination (no pupillary constriction to bright light) and pupils fixed in midposition or dilated 4 to 9 mm in diameter (Figure 14-1).

  —Absence of doll's eyes, that is, no compensatory eye movement in response to rapid rotation of the head to either side.

  —Absence of oculovestibular response on cold-caloric examination, wherein the tympanum is irrigated with ice water after the head has been tilted to 30° (to make the auditory canal vertical so that it will fill with cold water)—no eye deviation toward cold stimulus (Figure 14-2).

  —Absence of corneal reflex, that is, no blinking (Figure 14-3) when the cornea is touched (with a cotton swab or pledget).

  —Absence of gag reflex (Figure 14-4).

  —Absence of cough on suctioning or movement of the endotracheal tube.

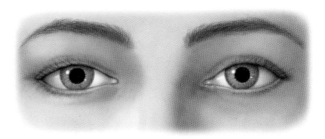

Figure 14-1. Pupils fixed and unresponsive to light.

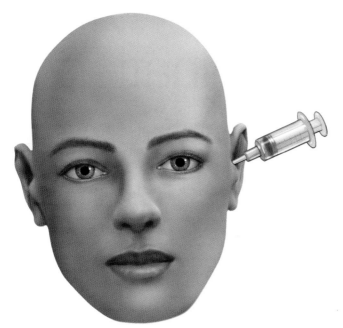

Figure 14-2. Eyes do not deviate toward cold water instilled into an auditory canal.

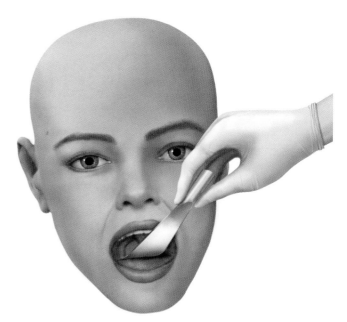

Figure 14-4. There is no gag or cough reflex.

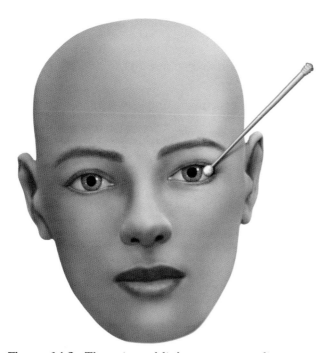

Figure 14-3. There is no blink response to direct corneal stimulation.

—Apnea test: Absence of spontaneous respiratory effort in response to a Pa_{CO_2} that is 60 mm Hg or 20 mm Hg greater than patient's normal baseline value.

—The test is typically performed after disconnection from the mechanical ventilator to avoid factitious breath sensing by ventilator sensors.

—The patient is typically preoxygenated with 100% oxygen prior to test to eliminate pulmonary stores of nitrogen and thereby reduce the possibility that the patient's hemoglobin oxygenation saturation will drop during apnea test (necessitating premature stopping of the test) prior to achievement of the threshold CO_2 level.

- Confirmatory tests

—Cerebral angiography should show no intracerebral filling from either the carotid or vertebral arteries, but the external carotid circulation should be patent.

—Electroencephalography should demonstrate no reactivity to somatosensory or audiovisual stimuli.

—Transcranial Doppler ultrasound should show absent diastolic flow with small early systolic peaks.

—Cerebral technetium scan should show the absence of intracranial filling (Figure 14-5).

- Brain death

—A patient meets the criteria for brain death following the performance of sequential (the interval is arbitrary, but a 6-hour interval is typical when the cause of coma is known, while a longer interval may be appropriate when the cause is undetermined) clinical examinations by a qualified examiner (typically an intensivist, neurologist, or neurosurgeon) consistent with brain death.

—The interval between sequential examinations may be shortened if there is a confirmatory test consistent with brain death.

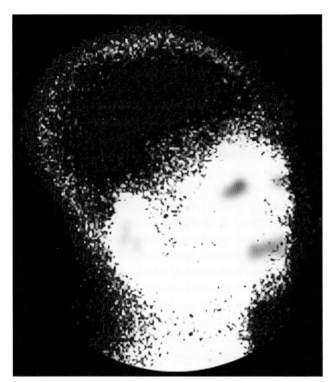

Figure 14-5. Blood flow is absent in the cranial vault when examined by cerebral scintigraphy (shown) or angiography.

 Clinical Pearls and Pitfalls

- Damage to the base of the pons, typically from a basilar artery embolism, can result in the development of the so-called locked-in syndrome, where the patient loses all voluntary movements with the exception of blinking and vertical eye movements.

- Guillain-Barré syndrome can involve all peripheral and cranial nerves and mimic brain death, but can be differentiated from it by the time course of the development of the disease which evolves over several days and by electrical and blood flow examinations.

- Hypothermia must be reversed prior to performance of the clinical examination to eliminate the confounding effects on the clinical examination.

- A variety of drugs including narcotics, benzodiazepines, tricyclic antidepressants, anticholinergics, and barbiturates can mimic brain death. It is prudent to administer reversal agents where the cause of coma is unknown and the agents are available (ie, naloxone, flumazenil). Alternatively, where drug levels are available, brain death should not be declared until the levels of these agents are subtherapeutic. If the serum level of a drug cannot be determined, declaration of brain death should not be done until several elimination half-lives have passed without change in the patient's examination.

- The cold-caloric oculocephalic examination can be confounded by wax or blood in the ear canal.

- Doll's eyes examination should not be performed if the cervical spine is unstable.

- Chronic obstructive pulmonary disease or sleep apnea may result in elevated baseline CO_2 retention, confounding the apnea examination.

- Certain spinal reflexes including spontaneous movements of the torso, arms, or toes may mimic volitional movements, but should be ignored if the clinical brain stem examination is consistent with brain death or confirmatory examinations are positive.

Suggested Reading

Quality Standards Committee of the American Academy of Neurology. Practice parameters for determining brain death in adults. *Neurology.* 1995;45: 1012–1014 (reconfirmed in 2003 and 2007).

Uniform Determination of Death Act.

Wijdicks EFM. Current concepts: the diagnosis of brain death. *N Engl J Med.* 2001;16:1215–1221.

CHAPTER 15

Intracranial Pressure Monitoring

 Introduction

The skull is a rigid container for the brain with a volume of about 1500 cc. The contents consist of brain parenchyma (80%), blood (10%), and cerebrospinal fluid (CSF) (10%). When injured, the brain swells, and because of the noncompliance of the skull, intracranial pressure (ICP) rises quickly. Treatment for ICP includes drugs that decrease the size of neurons (ie, mannitol, diuretics), drugs to put the brain to sleep (ie, barbiturates), hypothermia, brain resection, and craniectomy. The placement of a catheter in one of the ventricles permits both ICP monitoring and CSF drainage to reduce intracranial pressure. There are several alternative approaches to ICP monitoring, including intraparenchymal, subarachnoid, and epidural monitors. The latter tend to be less reliable than intraventricular monitors and preclude CSF drainage.

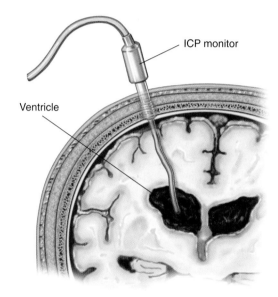

Figure 15-1. Diagram of ventriculostomy catheter in lateral ventricle.

 Definitions and Terms

- CPP: Cerebral perfusion pressure (mean arterial pressure minus ICP).
- CBF: Cerebral blood flow which is normally autoregulated should have a CPP value between 50 and 150 mm Hg.
- Ventriculostomy: Placement of a catheter in one of the brain ventricles through a small "burr hole" in the skull (Figure 15-1).
- Intraventricular monitor—considered to be the "gold standard" ICP monitor
  —Relatively high infection rate
  —Accurate and reliable
- Intraparenchymal monitor—a fiberoptic transducer placed in the brain parenchyma
  —Low infection rate
  —Tendency to "drift" over time

- Subarachnoid—fluid-coupled transduction of pressure on subarachnoid space
  —Low infection rate
  —Tendency to clog with debris
- Epidural—optical transduction of dural pressure
  —Tend to be inaccurate because pressure is damped
  —May be used in coagulopathic patients

 Techniques

- The following procedures should be performed prior to the intervention
  —Obtain informed consent.
  —Wash hands, gown, and glove, prepare, and drape site as described in Section I.
  —The hair surrounding the site should be clipped (Figure 15-2).

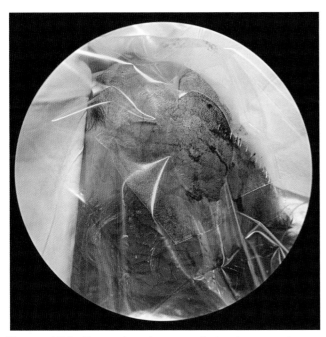

Figure 15-2. Draped and prepped site for ventriculostomy insertion.

■ Craniotomy

—The skin over the selected site is anesthetized with local anesthesia (typically the nondominant hemisphere).

—The insertion point is 1 cm anterior to the coronal suture in the mid-pupillary line

—A small incision is made in the skin down to the bone.

—A burr hole is made in the skull (Figure 15-3).

—The dura is then opened.

■ Ventriculostomy

—The catheter is passed through the dura and advanced, approximately, 7 cm (in an adult) toward the juncture of the lines passing from the incision point to the inner canthus of the ipsilateral eye and the from the tragus of the ear to the incision point toward the ipsilateral foramen of Monro (Figures 15-4 to15-7).

■ Correct intraventricular position can be verified by the free drainage of CSF through the catheter.

■ The intraventricular catheter is attached to a transducer to permit waveform and pressure monitoring,

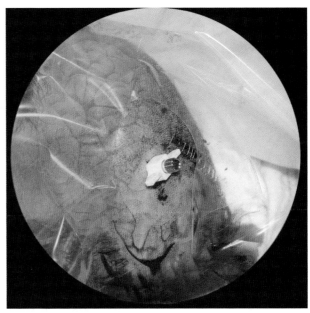

Figure 15-4. Bolt anchored (screwed into) skull and fitted for catheter placement.

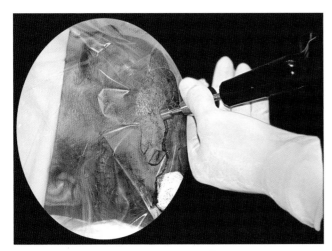

Figure 15-3. Twist-drill "burr-hole" procedure.

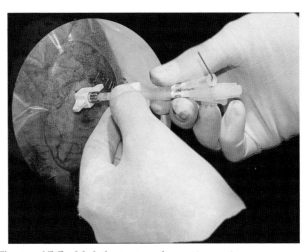

Figure 15-5. Multilumen catheter insertion.

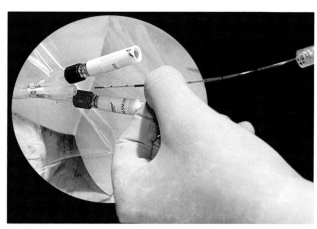

Figure 15-6. ICP transducer insertion.

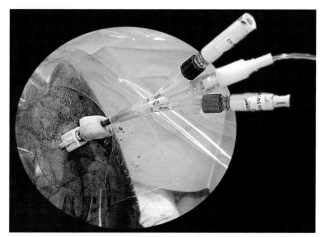

Figure 15-7. Completed procedure—with additional lumens for temperature and oxygen monitoring.

as well as stopcocked to allow intermittent CSF drainage.

- Normal ICP is less than 20 mm Hg.
- ICP should be treated (reduced) when ICP exceeds 20 mm Hg for a period greater than a few minutes.
- A secondary goal is to maintain a CPP between 60 and 75 mm Hg.

- Treatments for increased ICP include the following:
  —Hyperventilation
  —Diuresis
  —Head elevation
  —Sedation
  —Barbiturates
  —Hypertonic saline
  —Blood pressure control (to maintain CPP greater than 60 mm Hg and less than 120 mm Hg)
  —Maintenance of normothermia or cooling
  —Steroids
  —Ventilator adjustments (to reduce intrathoracic pressure)
  —CSF drainage (at 1-2 mL/min—usually through passive drainage)
  —Decompressive craniectomy

 Clinical Pearls and Pitfalls

- ICP monitoring is typically performed for brain-injured, comatose patients in whom a clinical examination cannot be performed.
- Additional indications include tumor, infection, mass lesions, cerebral edema, infarction, or hemorrhage.
- Contraindications include coagulopathy, severe hemodynamic instability, open wounds around planned site of insertion, immunosuppression, and small ventricles on computed tomographic (CT) or magnetic resonance imaging (MRI) scan.

Suggested Reading

Treggiari MM, Schultz N, Yanez ND, Romand JA. Role of intracranial pressure values and patterns in predicting outcome in traumatic brain injury: a systematic review. *Neurocrit Care.* 2007;6:104–112.

CHAPTER 16

Electroencephalography

 ## Introduction

The electroencephalogram (EEG) is used routinely in the intensive care unit (ICU) to evaluate patients for cortical electrical activity, and thereby to differentiate among various causes of coma, delirium, movement abnormalities, and identify brain death. In addition, EEG may be used to monitor depth of sedation. The EEG measures the summed voltage potentials (Figure 16-1) from a large number of neurons (not "brain waves"), and, depending on the number and placement of electrodes, can be used to localize certain pathological electrical processes in exactly the same way that an electrocardiogram (ECG) localizes injured cardiac muscle.

 ## Definitions and Terms

- Frequency: The measurement used to categorize several ranges of electrical activity found in the normal and abnormal brain:
  - Delta: High-amplitude, low-frequency waves seen in sleep
  - Theta: Low-frequency waves seen in younger children and meditation in adults—may be indicative of pathological activity, such as toxic encephalopathy
  - Alpha: Higher frequency range seen in relaxation and certain forms of coma
  - Beta: High frequencies seen during active thinking
- Epileptiform discharges: Rhythmic discharges seen focally or diffusely in patients with epilepsy.
- Diffuse slowing: Combination of delta and theta frequencies seen in many pathological states—when seen with preserved reactivity to external stimuli (ie, pain, sound); this pattern may have a better prognosis than when responsiveness is absent.
- Intermittent rhythmic delta activity: Pathological pattern that can be seen with metabolic, toxic, hypoxic, or other diffuse intracranial diseases.
- Burst suppression: High-voltage bursts of activity alternating with background suppression—seen in deep coma and pharmacologically induced coma.
- Bispectral index (BIS): A limited form of EEG analysis in which brain electrical activity is indexed to a dimensionless number between 0 and 100, wherein a value of 0 represents the absence of EEG activity and 100 is typical for an awake person—values between 40 and 60 are found in well-anesthetized patients.

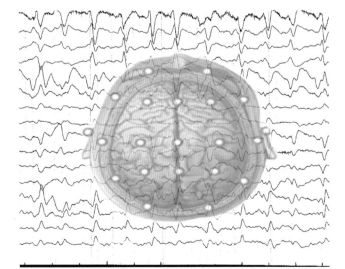

Figure 16-1. EEG tracing.

 ## Techniques

- EEG leads are placed circumferentially around the brain (Figures 16-2 and 16-3), as well as over the dome of the skull along coronal and saggital arcs—electrical activity is measured over specific areas of the brain (ie, frontal, temporal, cerebellar).
- EEG may be used in the delirious patient to determine whether abnormal electrical activity in the brain may be responsible for the delirious state.
- EEG is used as a diagnostic test in patients with diffuse or localized rhythmic movement to determine whether there is epileptic activity in the brain—the

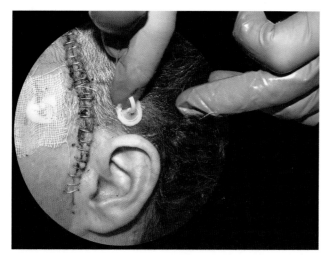

Figure 16-2. EEG lead placement (temporal).

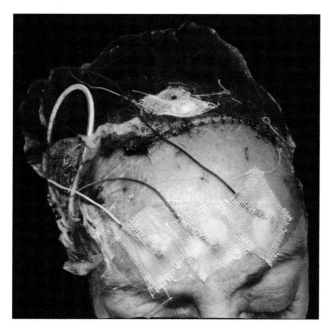

Figure 16-3. EEG lead placement (frontal).

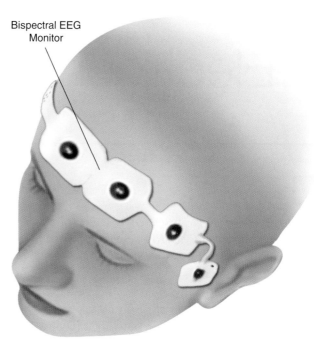

Bispectral EEG Monitor

Figure 16-4. Bispectral index monitoring with pads placed over forehead.

- BIS can be used to guide the administration of sedatives in the intensive care patient (Figure 16-4).

 Clinical Pearls and Pitfalls

- EEG is an electrical measurement and therefore subject to many of the artifacts common to any similar measurement, including artifact from poor connection, electrical interference, and muscle artifact.
- While EEG may be diagnostic in certain situations (ie, seizures), it is typically used in conjunction with structural studies (ie, radiographs) and the clinical examination to guide treatment and management.

 Suggested Reading

Vespa PM. Multimodality monitoring and telemonitoring in neurocritical care: from icrodialysis to robotic telepresence. *Curr Opin Crit Care.* 2005;11:133–138.
Young GB, Wang JT, Connolly JF. Prognostic determination in anoxic-ischemic and traumatic encephalopathies. *J Clin Neurophysiol.* 2004;21:379–390.

differential for rhythmic motor activity is long, but includes tremor, volitional movement, and shivering.

- EEG is used to establish prognosis in the comatose patient following a hypoxic event or cardiac arrest.
- EEG is used to guide pharmacological management of epileptic activity or intracranial hypertension.
- EEG is used as a confirmatory test in the diagnosis of brain death.

CHAPTER 17

Cerebral Oximetry

 ## Introduction

Cerebral oximetry is a noninvasive measurement of brain tissue oxygenation using near infrared spectroscopy. It can be used to show local brain tissue hypoxia or asymmetry in saturation between the two sides of the brain potentially indicating unilateral blood flow compromise.

 ## Definitions and Terms

- Near infrared spectroscopy: Light of multiple wavelengths (690-1100 nm) is passed through multiple tissue layers (skin, bone, brain) and reflected photons are measured by a receiver.
- Chromophores: Transmitted photons at certain wavelengths are absorbed by chromophores (ie, hemoglobin) in the tissue and the absorption will be a function of the degree of oxygen saturation of the hemoglobin.

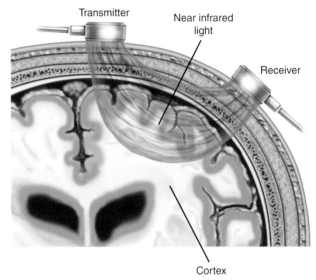

Figure 17-1. Diagram showing transmission of near infrared light and the arc it takes through brain tissue.

 ## Techniques

- Low-intensity, near infrared light is transmitted through a "source" applied (typically) to the forehead of a patient.
- Reflected/Transmitted light is measured at a point, approximately, 4 cm from the transmitter (Figure 17-1).
- Transmitter-receiver pairs are typically applied to each side of the forehead allowing comparison between left and right frontal lobe perfusion (Figure 17-2).

 ## Clinical Pearls and Pitfalls

- Transmitters and receivers should not be placed over skin with hair follicles (even shaven) because the follicles can absorb and alter light.
- Transcranial oximetry readings do not measure blood flow or oxygen uptake, and normal values may occur in the presence of active pathology if the pathology is not perfusion related.

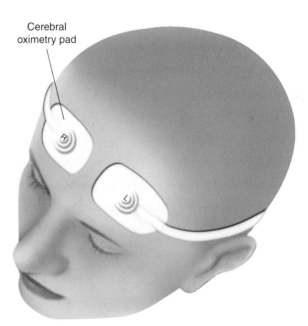

Figure 17-2. Oximetry pads applied to right and left forehead permitting comparison of oxygenation in north hemispheres.

- Cerebral oximetry shares many of the principals and applications of pulse oximetry.
- Electrocautery, movement, lead placement problems, and ambient light can all interfere with cerebral oximetry.

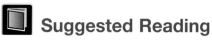 **Suggested Reading**

Casati A, Spreafico E, Putzu M, Fanelli G. New technology for noninvasive brain monitoring: continuous cerebral oximtery. *Minerva Anestesiol.* 2006;72:605–625.

CHAPTER 18

Direct Brain Tissue Oxygen Measurement

Introduction

Direct brain tissue oxygen measurement is used to determine whether treatments applied to the whole brain (ie, hyperventilation) are having beneficial or deleterious effects at the local (injured) tissue level.

Definitions and Terms

- $pBtO_2$: Partial pressure of oxygen in brain tissue
- TBI: Total brain injury
- DAI: Diffuse axonal injury
- SAH: Subarachnoid hemorrhage
- High $pBtO_2$: Values greater than 50 mm Hg
- Low $pBtO_2$: Values less than 20 mm Hg

Techniques

- The area of interest for tissue oxygen level monitoring is selected based on the underlying lesion.

  —TBI: The tip of the probe (Figure 18-1) is placed in or near the area of greatest injury on computed tomographic (CT) scan (ie, contusion, edema, subdural, extradural, intracerebral hematoma)—if there is no laterality, as in DAI, the probe should be placed on the right (to avoid left-sided speech centers) (Figure 18-2).

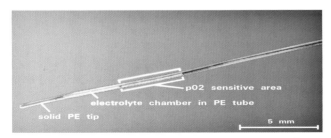

Figure 18-1. Brain tissue oxygen monitoring probe.

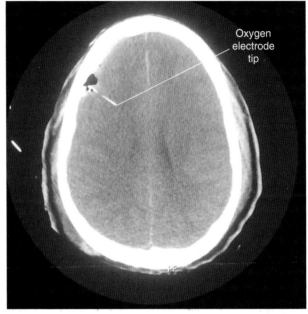

Figure 18-2. Heat scan showing probe in brain parenchyma in patient with cerebral edema.

  —SAH: The tip of the probe is placed in the area of expected vasospasm (ie, as indicated by aneurysm location or blood seen on CT scan).

  —Malignant stroke: Place on side of stroke as seen on CT scan.

  —The catheter may be placed in normal, but potentially at-risk, tissue.

- The preparation and catheter insertion are identical to the procedure described in Chapter 34, with the exception that the operator will select the site and advance the catheter into the area of interest as appropriate.

- $pBtO_2$ analysis:

  —High $pBtO_2$:

   • Increased delivery:

▪Due to hyperemia (potentially treat with hyperventilation)

• Decreased demand:

▪Due to hypothermia (may warrant warming)

▪Due to pharmacologic therapy (ie, sedatives, paralytics)

—Low $pBtO_2$:

• Increased demand:

▪Increased ICP (treat ICP with CSF drainage, pharmacotherapy)

▪Pain (treat with pain medication)

▪Shivering (treat pharmacologically, rewarm)

▪Agitation (sedate)

▪Seizures (pharmacotherapy)

▪Fever (treat with cooling, anti-inflammatory)

• Decreased delivery:

▪Hypotension, decreased perfusion (treat with fluids, pressors)

▪Hypovolemia (treat with fluids, blood products)

▪Anemia (treat with blood or blood replacement)

▪Hypoxia (increase FiO_2, increase PEEP [positive end-expiratory pressure], pulmonary toilet)

 ## Clinical Pearls and Pitfalls

▪Brain tissue oxygen monitoring is an advanced modality that will likely be used only in centers with the expertise to place the device, monitor, interpret, and treat brain tissue oxygen levels.

▪$pBtO_2$ will often be used as one of several brain monitoring modalities and the correct course of treatment may require a balancing act—that is, the administration of fluids or blood to a patient with increased ICP and decreased $pBtO_2$ in order to increase perfusion pressure

 ## Suggested Reading

van Santbrink H, Maas AI, Avezaat CJ. Continuous monitoring of partial pressure of brain tissue oxygen in patients with severe head injury. *Neurosurgery*. 1996;38:21–31.

CHAPTER 19

Jugular Venous Oximetry

Introduction

Jugular venous oximetry is a method of analyzing the balance between oxygen supply and demand to the brain. The oxygen saturation of blood draining from the brain into the jugular bulb is continuously measured providing an indirect measure of oxygen extraction by the brain.

Definitions and Terms

- Jugular venous bulb: Dilation of the internal jugular vein in the jugular fossa of the temporal bone
- $SjvO_2$: Jugular venous oxygen saturation
- $AVjDO_2$: Arteriovenous jugular oxygen content $(Hgb \times 1.34[SaO_2 - SjO_2] + 0.003[PaO_2 - PvO_2])$
- CaO_2: Artcrial oxygen content saturation
- $CjvO_2$: Jugular venous oxygen saturation
- CeO_2: Cerebral extraction of oxygen $(SaO_2 [\%] - SjvO_2 [\%])$
- $CMRO_2$: Cerebral metabolic rate of oxygen
- O_2ER: Global cerebral oxygen extraction ratio
- CMRL: Cerebral metabolic rate of lactate
- AVDL: Arteriovenous difference of lactate
- LOI: Lactate Index $(AVDL/AVDO_2 [ischemia > 0.08])$

Techniques

- Patient consent should be obtained prior to performance of the procedure and the site should be prepped and draped as described in Section 1 (Figure 19-1).
- The jugular vein is cannulated in the usual fashion, and the $SjvO_2$ catheter is threaded retrograde until it reaches the roof of the jugular bulb, at which point some resistance will be felt (usually 13-15 cm from the skin).

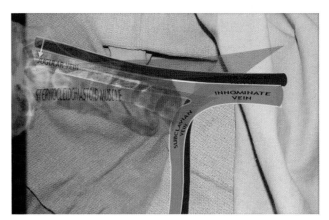

Figure 19-1. Jugular venous tip placement.

- The catheter should then be withdrawn approximately 1 cm and monitoring initiated.
- A skull x-ray is performed after insertion to verify correct position of the catheter tip.
- Normal $SjvO_2$ is between 55% to 70%.
- Normal $AVjDO_2$ is 3.5 to 8 mL/dL.
- Normal CeO_2 is 24% to 42%.
- $SjvO_2$
  —Greater than 75% implies "luxury perfusion"
  —Less than 50% represents hypoperfusion
  —Less than 40% represents ischemia

Clinical Pearls and Pitfalls

- The signal quality indicator is a measure of the quality of the signal received at the tip of the catheter; poor signal quality may indicate clotting at the tip or that the tip is up against the vessel wall—the catheter should be flushed and/or the head repositioned.
- Normal $SjvO_2$ are possible even in the face of significant brain pathology:
  —Focal ischemia may not be apparent.
  —Venous drainage may be asymmetric.

—Infratentorial (brainstem, cerebellum) injuries are not monitored by jugular venous drainage.

- Jugular venous monitoring is contraindicated in coagulopathy, impaired venous drainage, neck trauma, tracheostomy (risk of infection), cervical spine injuries (difficulty of cannulation), and local infection.

 Suggested Reading

Woodman T, Robertson CS. Jugular venous oxygen saturation monitoring. In: Narayan RK, Wilberger JE, Povlishock JT eds. *Neurotrauma*. New York: McGraw-Hill; 1996. 519–537; Chap 36.

CHAPTER 20

Cerebral Microdialysis

 Introduction

Cerebral microdialysis involves placement of a small catheter with a semipermeable membrane in the parenchyma of the brain, so that a dialysate fluid can be instilled into the catheter, allowed to equilibrate and withdrawn for analysis (Figure 20-1). Neurochemical levels such as lactate, pyruvate, glucose, and glutamate can then be measured to determine metabolic and neurotransmitter activity in the area of interest.

 Definitions and Terms

- Microdialysis: A technique used to determine the chemical composition of extracellular fluid in a tissue/organ of interest.
- Lactate: Chemical by-product of anaerobic metabolism.
- Glutamate: Amino acid and excitatory neurotransmitter.
- Glycerol: A marker of cell membrane breakdown.

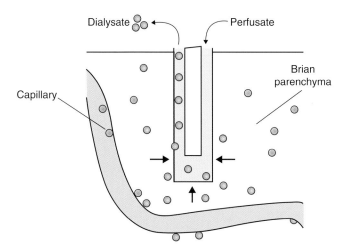

Figure 20-1. Diagram showing microdialysis catheter in brain parenchyma adjacent to capillary, and molecules of interest (ie, pyruvate, lactate, glutamate, glucose, glycerol) entering dialysate.

 Techniques

- The insertion technique for cerebral microdialysis is similar to the technique described for ventriculostomy:
  —Shave and prepare insertion site
  —Small skin incision and burr hole
  —Incise dura and advance catheter into area of interest
- The tip of the catheter can be positioned in various areas depending on the nature of the underlying lesion, but microdialysis is primarily used to monitor neurochemical changes in tissue at risk for secondary injury following a primary neurological event:
  —The catheter may be placed in the nondominant hemisphere to monitor global cerebral events in diffuse axonal injury.
  —The catheter may be implanted in the less injured hemisphere of a brain-injured patient to determine the effect of whole brain interventions, such as hyperventilation on vulnerable tissue.
  —The catheter may be positioned in the penumbral area around infarcted or contused brain to evaluate the effects of treatments on the at-risk tissue surrounding irretrievably injured brain.
  —The catheter may be placed in an area of tissue perfused by arteries susceptible to vasospasm to monitor the effects of interventions designed to treat vasospasm.

 Clinical Pearls and Pitfalls

- Low glucose levels in microdialysate indicates reduced cerebral glucose supply and/or cerebral hypoxia and ischemia.
- An increase in the lactate-pyruvate ratio may result from hypoxia-ischemia, reduction in cellular redox state, mitochondrial dysfunction, or low cerebral glucose supply and is probably the most reliable indicator of local ischemia.
- Increased glycerol level indicates hypoxia/ischemia and cell membrane degradation, although it may be due to systemic events rather than local cell breakdown.

■Increased glutamate levels have traditionally been suspected of a causal role in "excitotoxicity," wherein glutamate release after injury, but there is significant variability in glutamate both within and among patients with brain injury.

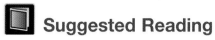 **Suggested Reading**

Tisdall MM, Smith M. Cerebral microdialysis: research technique or clinical tool. *BJA.* 2006;97:18–25.

CHAPTER 21

Transcranial Doppler Examination

 Introduction

Transcranial Doppler (TCD) ultrasound examination of blood flow velocity through the brain can be used to detect cerebral arterial vasospasm, steno-occlusive disease of the cerebral arteries, or the absence of blood flow (in the determination of brain death).

 Definitions and Terms

- Doppler ultrasound: A technique based on the principles of sound travel and reflectance in tissues—transmitted sound waves change their frequency when they come into contact with moving blood cells and the frequency change is known as the Doppler effect.

- Blood flow velocity: Measurement of the speed (Figure 21-1) and direction of blood flow (as distinct from total blood flow).

- Continuous wave Doppler: Continuous measurement of sound pitch changes relating to blood flow velocity through vessels, around obstructions, or through narrowings.

- Duplex Doppler: Provides a picture of the vessels and information about the speed and direction of blood flow in the vessels.

- Color flow Doppler: Velocities are mapped into colors and overlaid on the image of the blood vessels.

- Acoustic window: A portion of the skull that permits transmission and reception of ultrasound through the skull—the temporal, transorbital, suboccipital, and submandibular windows are typically used.

 Techniques

- The probe is applied lightly to the skin over the acoustic window using ultrasound gel to improve contact and sound wave transmission (Figure 21-2).

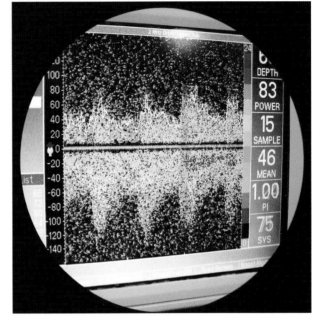

Figure 21-1. Color map of blood flow velocities in an artery of interest.

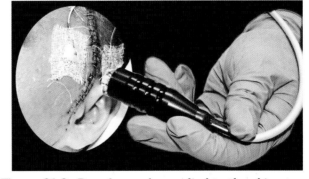

Figure 21-2. Doppler probe applied to the skin over the temporal acoustic window.

- Indications
  - Evaluation of intracranial vascular disease
  - Monitoring of vasospasm (increased blood flow velocity through narrowed vessels)

—Detection of cerebral emboli

—Evaluation of vertebrobasilar vascular disease

—Detection of arteriovenous malformations

 TCD temporal bone windows are not as good in females as in males.

■ Arterial velocities increase in anemia, as viscosity decreases.

■ Arterial velocities are increased in fever.

 ## Clinical Pearls and Pitfalls

■ Normal cerebral arterial velocities decrease with age, which is phenomenon related to decreasing cardiac output.

Suggested Reading

Katz ML, Alexandrov AV. *A Practical Guide to Transcranial Doppler Examinations*. Littleton, CO: Summer Publishing Company; 2003.

CHAPTER 22

Portable Computerized Axial Tomography Scanning

 ## Introduction

While not widely accessible, portable computerized axial tomography (CT) scanning (Figure 22-1) has become available commercially and is ideal for the intensive care unit (ICU) patient, who may be at risk during transportation to and from the remotely located CT scanner.

 ## Definitions and Terms

- Neurological emergency: Unexplained change in mental status, obtundation, or neurological deficit

 ## Techniques

- CT scan with or without contrast is the standard approach to the radiographic determination of intracranial anatomy and pathology.

- Noncontrast CT can be used to reveal intracranial hemorrhage, large cerebrovascular events, skull trauma and evaluate ventricular size.

- Contrast enhancement is used to evaluate specific lesions which will become more apparent to the presence of contrast in the blood flowing through the lesion, that is, infection or tumor.

 ## Clinical Pearls and Pitfalls

- Contrast dye may be unnecessary for certain patients and contraindicated for other (ie, renal insufficiency, contrast dye allergy).

- Contrast dye can cause afferent arteriolar vasospasm in the kidney, and patients with certain conditions (ie, diabetes, myeloma, renal insufficiency, dehydration, and congestive heart failure) are at increased risk.

- Prophylactic hydration reduces the risk of contrast nephropathy, as may prophylactic administration of N-acetylcysteine.

 ## Suggested Reading

Teichgraber UKM, Pinkernelle J, Jurgensen J, Ricke J, Kaisers U. Portable computed tomography performed on the intensive care unit. *Intensive Care Med.* 2003;29:491–495.

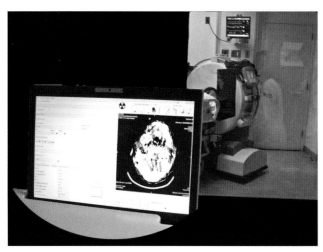

Figure 22-1. CT scanning console in the foreground, with an ICU patient in CT gantry in the background.

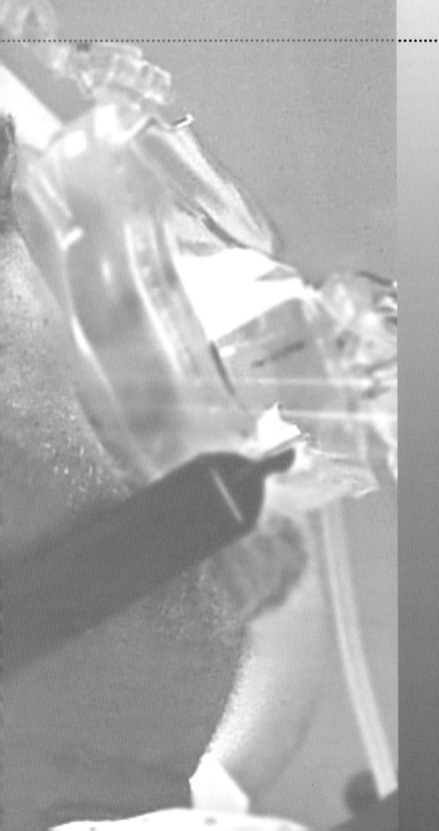

SECTION III

Thoracic and
Respiratory
Procedures

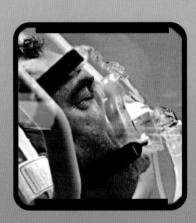

CHAPTER 23

Emergency Airway Cart

 Introduction

The emergency airway cart (Figure 23-1) is designed to be immediately available in the intensive care setting equipped with a variety of equipment that can be used to facilitate endotracheal intubation or alternative airway management approaches (ie, percutaneous airway) when standard approaches have failed.

 Definitions and Terms

- ETT: Endotracheal tube.
- Difficult airway: The clinical situation in which a skilled operator experiences difficulty with face mask ventilation of the upper airway, difficulty with tracheal intubation, or both.

- LMA: Laryngeal mask airway.
- TTJV: Transtracheal jet ventilation.
- Surgical airway: Percutaneous tracheal intubation—techniques include cricothyroidotomy and tracheostomy.
- Retrograde intubation: Transtracheal passage of a wire through the vocal cords and into the pharynx where it is retrieved by operator, which is then used to guide (pull) the ETT into correct position in the trachea.
- Combined esophageal/tracheal tube: A tube designed so that the distal tip sits in and occludes the esophagus, while proximal orifices are used to permit tracheal ventilation.

 Techniques

- Emergency airway cart equipment may include:
  —Rigid laryngoscope blades of alternate design and size from those routinely used; this may include a rigid fiberoptic
  —Laryngoscope
  —Tracheal tubes of assorted sizes
  —Masks of various sizes
  —Tracheal tube guides, examples include (but are not limited to) semirigid stylets, ventilating tube changer, light wands, and forceps designed to manipulate the distal portion of the tracheal tube
  —LMAs of assorted sizes
  —Flexible fiberoptic intubation equipment
  —Retrograde intubation equipment
  —At least one device suitable for emergency noninvasive airway ventilation, examples include (but are not limited to) an esophageal tracheal tube, a hollow jet ventilation stylet, and a transtracheal jet ventilator
  —Equipment suitable for emergency invasive airway access (ie, cricothyrotomy)
  —An exhaled CO_2 detector

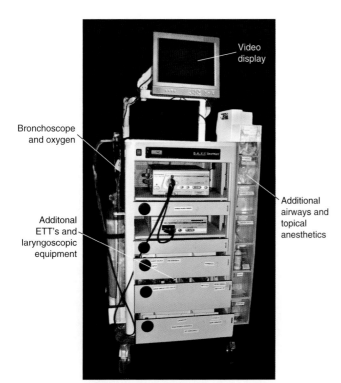

Figure 23-1. Difficult airway cart.

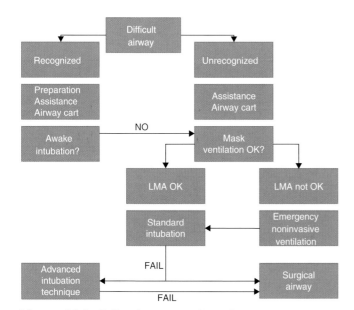

Figure 23-2. Difficult airway algorithm.

■The American Society of Anesthesiology has published a difficult airway algorithm (Figure 23-2) that describes a pathway for handling unexpected problems with ventilation and intubation of the anesthetized patient, which is equally applicable to the intensive care patient.

■In the event of difficulties with ventilation:

—Consider or attempt placement of an LMA and ventilation.

—Call for help.

—Attempt endotracheal intubation.

—Attempt emergency noninvasive ventilation using:

• Esophageal/tracheal tube

• TTJV

—In the event that the preceding measures are unsuccessful, proceed to surgical airway.

■If mask ventilation is adequate and initial intubation unsuccessful.

—Attempt endotracheal intubation using alternative approaches including:

• Alternate laryngoscope blade

• Reposition head

• LMA placed as a bridge to intubation, where bronchoscopy is performed through LMA, and ETT threaded over bronchoscope

• Bronchoscopic intubation with ETT threaded over bronchoscope

• Retrograde intubation

—In the event that the preceding measures are unsuccessful, proceed to surgical airway.

 Clinical Pearls and Pitfalls

■Prior to performance of any airway procedure, a quick examination should be performed to evaluate airway anatomy and determine the potential for difficulties with intubation.

■If time permits, and the airway appears to be difficult, the emergency airway cart should be brought to the bedside.

■Call for assistance as soon as it becomes apparent that difficulties are likely—this may include respiratory therapy, additional skilled airway operators, and/or operators who can perform a surgical airway if needed.

■Consider carefully before administration of agents that obtund airway reflexes or paralyze the patient, that is, could the procedure be performed with the patient awake?

■When a difficult airway is encountered, do not engage in techniques with which you lack familiarity (i.e. retrograde cannulation).

 Suggested Reading

Practice guideline for management of the difficult airway. *Anesthesiology*. 2003;98:1269–1277.

CHAPTER 24

Bag-Mask Ventilation

Introduction

Bag-mask ventilation is often used as a way to supplement or replace spontaneous patient respiratory attempts prior to endotracheal intubation. Various anatomic issues (ie, excess soft tissue, large tongue) may necessitate the insertion of an artificial airway to permit bag-mask ventilation.

Definitions and Terms

- Resuscitation bag: Typically a self-reinflating bag with standard connectors for oxygen administration and connection to a face mask and/or endotracheal tube connector (Figure 24-1)

 —Valved to separate inhaled gas from exhaled gas

 —Permits ventilation with room air in the absence of a supplemental oxygen supply

 —Permits ventilation with oxygen enriched gas when connected to an oxygen supply

- Face mask: A soft cuff mask designed to fit over the nose and mouth of a patient with a seal permitting positive pressure ventilation without gas leak (Figure 24-2)

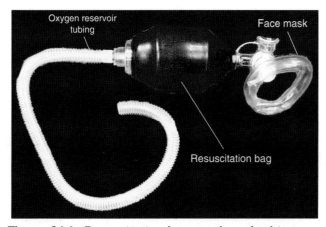

Figure 24-1. Resuscitation bag, mask, and tubing.

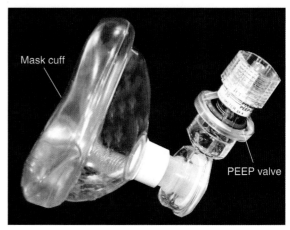

Figure 24-2. Face mask with attached PEEP valve.

 —Various sized masks permit selection of the appropriate size for a given patient.

 —Masks are equipped with a universal connector for attachment to resuscitation bag and/or ventilator tubing.

 —Transparent plastic masks permit recognition of vomitus if the patient regurgitates.

Techniques

- Select appropriate mask for patient's face size.
- Apply mask to face over nose and mouth with left hand.
- The thumb should be above the endotracheal tube connector and the index finger below, with the remaining fingers spread along mandible (Figure 24-3).
- The bag should be compressed in coordination with the patient's inspiratory effort, if present or at a rate between 10 and 20 breaths/min if patient efforts absent.
- The chest should be inspected for appropriate rise and fall with bag compressions.
- The abdomen should be inspected for enlargement to determine whether the stomach is being inflated with bag compressions.

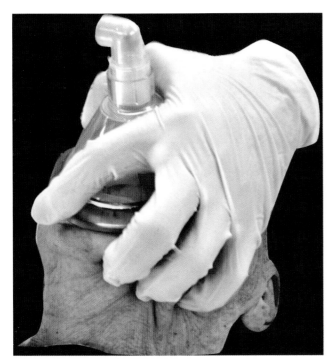

Figure 24-3. Hand position on mask.

 Clinical Pearls and Pitfalls

- Patients with certain kinds of facial anatomy (ie, beard, edentulous, excess soft tissue) are difficult to ventilate with a mask.

- The mask can be rocked in various directions to enhance the seal.

- If it becomes apparent that the stomach is inflating, an artificial airway should be placed, and Sellick's maneuver performed (see Chapter 27) to compress esophagus during ventilation—the stomach should then be decompressed following endotracheal intubation if applicable.

 Suggested Reading

Ortega R, Mehio AK, Woo A, Hafez DH. Positive-pressure ventilation with a face mask and a bag-valve device. *N Engl J Med*. 2007;357:e4.

CHAPTER 25

Noninvasive Ventilation

 Introduction

Noninvasive ventilation is a ventilatory technique in which a patient receives ventilatory assistance without the need for endotracheal intubation or a tracheostomy. While both negative and positive pressure ventilation are possible, the latter will be the focus of this chapter.

 Definitions and Terms

- Noninvasive positive pressure ventilation (NPPV): Positive pressure ventilation delivered via nasal or full face mask using volume, pressure, bilevel positive airway pressure (BIPAP), or continuous positive pressure (CPAP) modes.

- CPAP: Positive pressure is applied through the mask at one pressure—CPAP is typically used for patient with upper airway obstruction to open collapsed airways.

- BIPAP: A ventilatory mode in which CPAP is supplied cycling between a higher and lower pressure at a regular rate—BIPAP is typically used to reduce the work of breathing and augment alveolar ventilation.
  —Timed mode: Ventilator cycles regularly between high and low pressures and patient can breathe at each.
  —Spontaneous mode (ie, pressure support): Patient inspiration triggers application of the higher pressure.

- Nasal mask: A mask applied over the nose, leaving the mouth uncovered—may be adequate for CPAP administration in diseases such as sleep apnea.

- Face mask: A mask applied over the nose and mouth—often preferred in acute respiratory failure, because most patients in this situation breathe primarily through the mouth.

- ARF: Acute respiratory failure.
- CHF: Congestive heart failure.

 Techniques

- There are a variety of potential indications for the application of NPPV.
  —Respiratory insufficiency in patients with COPD
  —Respiratory insufficiency in patients with ARF
  —Respiratory insufficiency following extubation
  —Respiratory insufficiency with asthma
  —Respiratory insufficiency in patient with CHF and pulmonary edema
  —Respiratory insufficiency in patients with restrictive lung diseases and neuromuscular disorders

- There are a variety of contraindications to NPPV.
  —Status post respiratory arrest
  —Facial trauma
  —Agitation, claustrophobia, lack of patient cooperation
  —Excessive secretions
  —High risk of regurgitation and aspiration
  —Hemodynamic lability
  —Decreased/impaired mental status
  —Severe hypoxemia

- Patient preparation.
  —Select appropriate mask (nasal vs. face) and size to patient.
  —Secure mask to patient using circumferential straps around the head.
  —Adjust for maximal patient comfort (Figure 25-1).
  —Elevate head of bed to 45°.
  —Selected ventilatory mode.
  —Titrate ventilatory and oxygen support to achieve desired goals (Figure 25-2).
  —Monitor respiratory rate, tidal volume, and pulse oximetry.

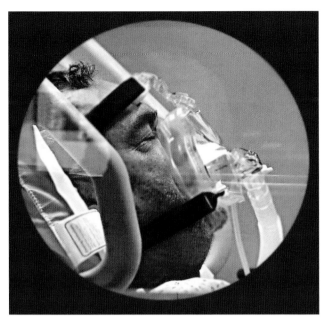

Figure 25-1. Full face mask NPPV.

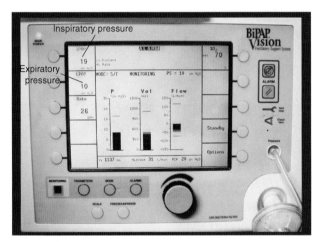

Figure 25-2. BIPAP ventilator with inspiratory and expiratory settings.

 Clinical Pearls and Pitfalls

▪Skillful mask selection and fitting will maximize ventilatory support.

▪Certain patients are difficult to fit properly due to anatomic reasons (ie, beard, edentulousness).

▪The mask should be strapped securely but not so tightly as to cause discomfort or skin breakdown.

▪Deteriorating hemodynamics or blood gases following initiation of NPPV warrant endotracheal intubation and standard mechanical ventilation.

▪Many patients will be benefited by cycled NPPV, with periods of support interrupted by support free intervals during which they may eat and/or communicate unimpeded.

 Suggested Reading

Garpestad E, Brennan J, Hill, NS. Noninvasive ventilation for critical care. *Chest.* 2007;132:711–720.

CHAPTER 26

Laryngeal Mask Airway

 ## Introduction

The laryngeal mask airway (LMA) is used widely in the operating room for airway management during anesthesia, but is also recognized as a "rescue" technique in emergency airway management. An LMA is a wide bore airway with a standard tube connector at one end (Figure 26-1) and a cuffed, (inverted) teardrop-shaped distal end (Figures 26-2 to 26-3) designed to sit over the larynx with the cuff inflated (Figure 26-4), thereby isolating the airway from the esophagus and oropharynx and preventing aspiration.

 ## Definitions and Terms

- Mask: Inverted teardrop shaped concave mask with central fenestrations to tube and a circumferential compliant cuff designed to seal the mask against the larynx with a low-pressure seal
- Tube: The tubular conduit of the LMA between the mask and the connector
- Intubating LMA: A special variant of the LMA designed to facilitate emergency ventilation and airway management, followed by bronchoscopy and

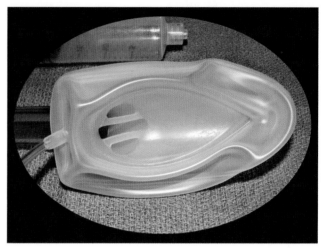

Figure 26-2. Laryngeal mask with teardrop shape, cuff deflated and showing fenestrated air passage.

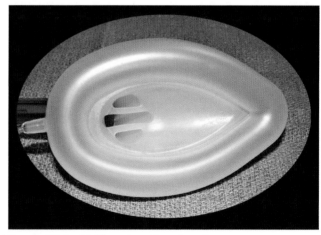

Figure 26-3. LMA with inflated cuff.

passage of a standard endotracheal tube through the LMA and over the bronchoscope

 ## Techniques for Laryngeal Mask Airway Insertion

- Indications for the use of an LMA in emergency airway management

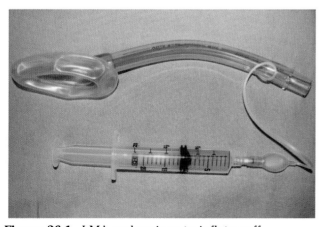

Figure 26-1. LMA and syringe to inflate cuff.

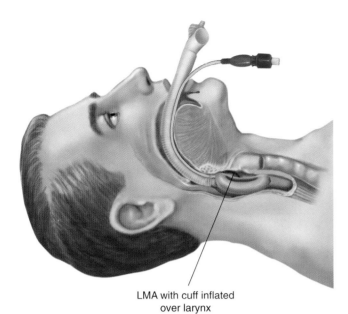

LMA with cuff inflated
over larynx

Figure 26-4. Graphic showing LMA cuff in correct position covering tracheal inlet.

—For emergency *ventilation* when mask ventilation is unsuccessful (ie, in the patient with a difficult airway)

—Emergency airway access when endotracheal intubation is unsuccessful

—Conduit for fiberoptic intubation

▪Preparation: Prior to LMA insertion, the universal protocol (Chapter 3) should be performed including timeout, consent, and equipment setup

　—Equipment: Ensure the availability and functioning of all required equipment including:

　　• Oxygen source

　　• Functioning suction circuit

　　• Large bore (ie, Yankauer) suction device during procedure

　　• Selection of appropriately sized LMA tubes with competent cuffs (where relevant)

　　• Self-inflating ventilation bag with attached oxygen feed

　　• Selection of face masks

　　• Selection of oral and nasal airways

　　• Pulse oximeter to monitor patient oxygenation during procedure

　　• End-tidal CO_2 detector to determine correct tube placement following procedure

　　• Bronchoscope and endotracheal tubes if LMA insertion is intended as a temporizing measure prior to endotracheal intubation

　　• Mechanical ventilator (while a mechanical ventilator is not necessary for performance of the procedure, most patients will be placed on a mechanical ventilator immediately following intubation)

　—Personnel

　　• Ensure the availability of skilled assistance during performance of procedure including respiratory therapist, nurse to monitor patient during performance of procedure and assist in procedure.

　—Patient

　　• The patient should be preoxygenated prior to procedure, if possible, to minimize the possibility of desaturation during the procedure—this is typically done with a period of enriched oxygen breathing prior to endotracheal intubation.

　　• Positioning: The patient should be placed in the "sniffing" position with head flexed on torso, and neck extended, to optimize airway alignment (this can be done by putting the patient's head on a small pillow or by placing a towel roll behind the patient's neck). Elevate the head of the bed where possible.

　　• Ensure the availability of a free flowing intravenous catheter for medication administration.

▪LMA selection and preparation

　—LMA come in a variety of sizes, the standard size is the size 4; a size 3 can be used for small adults and a size 5 for larger adults or in situations where the size 4 does not seal adequately following cuff inflation.

　—The LMA mask and cuff should be well lubricated prior to insertion.

　—Cuff patency should be verified and the cuff should then be fully deflated.

　—A syringe of the appropriate size should be attached to the LMA or immediately available—a size 4 LMA holds approximately 30 cc of air, whereas a size 5 holds 40 cc of air.

▪LMA insertion

　—The operator stands behind the patient as with endotracheal intubation (Figure 26-5).

　—The LMA mask and flattened cuff are advanced into the patient's open mouth along the hard palate, past the uvula and into the hypopharynx.

　—A finger can be used to guide the mask into the hypopharynx (Figure 26-6), or the jaw distracted anteriorly as the mask passes into the hypopharynx and over the larynx—this minimizes the likelihood that the mask and cuff will fold over, force the

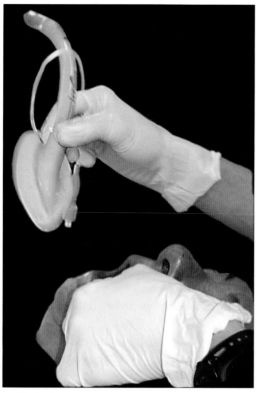

Figure 26-5. Operator opening mouth prior to LMA insertion.

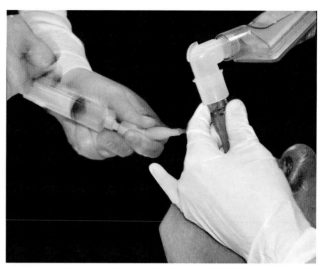

Figure 26-7. Cuff inflation after LMA insertion.

epiglottis over the cords or enter and occlude the airway.

—The cuff is then inflated (Figures 26-7 to 26-8) to the recommended volume (overinflation may cause misplacement or obstruction).

—Correct tube position is confirmed by positive pressure ventilation with audible breath sounds and end-tidal CO_2 detection.

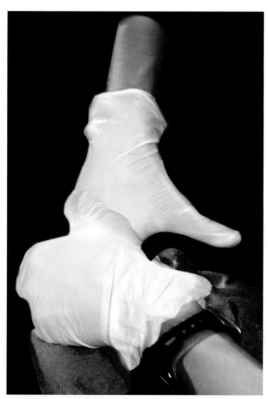

Figure 26-6. LMA placement where operator uses right hand to seat cuff.

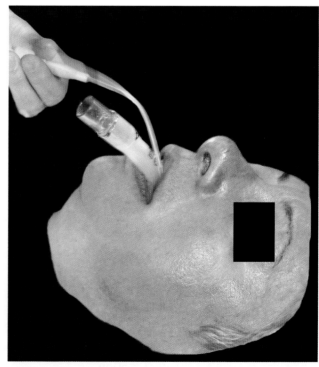

Figure 26-8. LMA in correct position.

—If ventilation is unsuccessful, the LMA can be repositioned or a larger LMA can be substituted.

- Contraindications to LMA insertion, which should be considered relative considerations when LMA is used as an emergency airway management technique

 —Obesity or pregnancy

 —Massive facial or airway injuries

 ## Clinical Pearls and Pitfalls

- The LMA should be included in emergency airway carts and may be included in standard airway boxes.
- Lubricant should only be applied to the cuff and back of the mask, not the laryngeal surface.

- A poorly lubricated LMA is more likely to fold on itself during passage.
- The LMA should be secured with a bite block in the mouth and taped to prevent dislodgement during subsequent airway management (ie, bronchoscopy).

 ## Suggested Reading

Langeron O, Amour J, Vivien B, Aubrun F. Clinical review: management of difficult airways. *Crit Care*. 2006;10:243.

Cook TM, Hommers C. New airways for resuscitation. *Resuscitation*. 2006;69:371–387.

CHAPTER 27

Oral Endotracheal Intubation

 Introduction

Endotracheal intubation is the definitive way to secure an airway in a patient with respiratory insufficiency, cardiopulmonary insufficiency, or neurological compromise. This chapter will discuss oral and nasal endotracheal intubation.

 Definitions and Terms

- Airway: Conduit through which gas passes between the atmosphere and the lungs, including the oropharynx, nasopharynx, hypopharynx, trachea, or an artificial airway such as an endotracheal tube (ETT).

- ETT: An artificial airway usually inserted through the mouth or nose into the trachea (Figure 27-1). While a variety of variants are available for specialty uses, the typical ETT has the following features:

—Made of flexible, clear plastic material.

—Equipped with a standard-sized (universal) 15 mm connector at the proximal end, which ensures

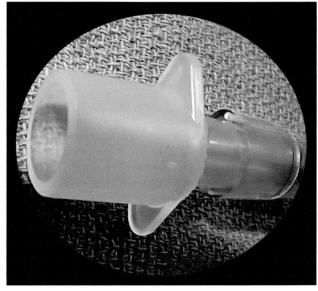

Figure 27-2. A standard (universal) ETT connector.

compatibility with all ventilator circuits and ventilation bags (Figure 27-2).

—Having an opaque stripe along the length of the tubing to facilitate tube location on chest x-ray.

—Beveled tip to facilitate passage through vocal cords.

—Length markers to assist in correct placement of ETT.

—ETTs may or may not be equipped with an inflatable cuff just proximal to the distal tip of the tube which can be inflated to sequester the trachea from the hypopharynx—pediatric ETTs are typically uncuffed to maximize the available diameter of the tube for gas passage, whereas adult tubes are typically cuffed.

—Cuffed ETTs are often equipped with a "Murphy eye," which is a side vent just proximal to the distal end of the tube, designed to allow an alternative air passage in the event that the distal tip was

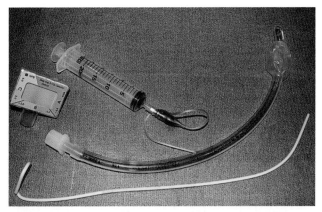

Figure 27-1. A standard ETT with a syringe attached to the "pilot balloon" for cuff inflation, as well as a malleable stylet to form the tube during insertion and an end-tidal C_2 detector.

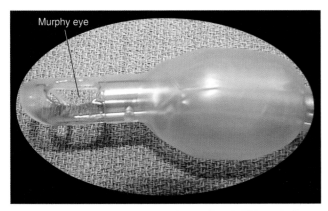

Figure 27-3. The distal tip of a cuffed ETT with the cuff inflated, beveled tip and Murphy eye (see text).

occluded by contact with the tracheal wall or a plug (Figure 27-3).

- Laryngoscope (Figure 27-4): One of a variety of tools designed to allow an operator to open and align the oral pharynx and hypopharynx, and illuminate the vocal cords, thereby permitting insertion of an oral ETT under direct visualization.

- Direct laryngoscopy: The act of using a laryngoscope to visualize the airway—as compared with indirect laryngoscopy using either a mirror or fiberoptic laryngoscopy. The latter procedures are typically performed for diagnostic reasons.

- Oral entotracheal intubation: Placement of the distal tip of an ETT in the trachea, typically using direct laryngoscopy, although the procedure can be performed using a fiberoptic bronchoscope to locate the airway and subsequently threading the ETT over the bronchoscope into the trachea.

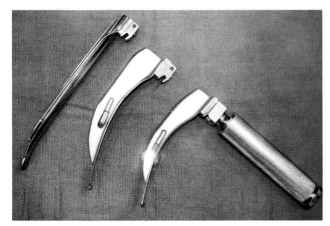

Figure 27-4. A laryngoscope with a variety of blades.

- Nasal endotracheal intubation: Placement of the distal tip of an ETT into the trachea after passage of the ETT through the nose, nasopharynx and hypopharynx. The ETT can be passed blindly using breath sounds as a locator or alternatively threaded over a bronchoscope.

 ## Techniques

- Indications for endotracheal intubation in the ICU

—Respiratory insufficiency with hypercarbia and or hypoxia

- Hypercarbia: Commonly due to hypoventilation, airway obstruction, or increased CO_2 production

- Hypoxia: Inadequate systemic oxygenation that cannot be managed with supplemental inhaled oxygen

—Airway obstruction: Typically due to airway laxity (ie, snoring), soft tissue swelling (ie, after trauma, surgery)

—Patient inability to clear secretions or "protect" airway with cough: due to cerebral vascular event, head trauma, drug, or alcohol intoxication

—Catastrophic cardiac or neurological event: cardiac arrest, or increased intracranial pressure, coma

 ## Techniques for Endotracheal Intubation

- Oral endotracheal intubation:

—Once the decision to intubate has been made, several additional factors need to be considered including the urgency of the intervention, the patient's current mental status, the degree to which the anatomy of the patient's airway may interfere with procedure, and whether or not the patient is at risk for regurgitation during the procedure (ie, full stomach).

- Urgency: If the patient is apneic, intubation must be performed immediately, whereas if the patient is relatively hypercapneic or hypoxic, the procedure can be performed with more deliberation.

- Mental status: A patient who is relatively obtunded may be intubated with no to minimal sedation, whereas an awake and agitated patient typically will need to be sedated and paralyzed to perform direct laryngoscopy.

- Airway anatomy: While a full discussion of the anatomic issues associated with oral intubation is beyond the scope of this text, the following anatomic features are indicative of the potential for difficulties with intubation that can complicate the procedure:

- Small jaw
- "Buck" teeth
- Stiff neck
- Edentulous mouth
- Relatively anterior larynx
- Tongue or airway soft tissue swelling

• Regurgitation: Most emergency intubations should be performed with the assumption that the patient has a full stomach and the following precautionary measures taken where feasible:

- Gastric emptying prior to endotracheal intubation (ie, if a nasogastric tube is in place).
- Elevated head of bed during procedure: To minimize passive regurgitation.
- Performance of "Sellick's maneuver" (compressing larynx against esophagus) during laryngoscopy.
- Ensure immediate access to large bore (ie, Yankauer) suction device during procedure.
- "Rapid sequence" intubation: Where the patient breathes an oxygen-rich air mixture prior to procedure and is then sedated and paralyzed in rapid sequence and immediately intubated without intervening positive pressure ventilation.

—Preparation: Prior to endotracheal intubation, the universal protocol (Chapter 3) should be performed including timeout, consent, and equipment setup.

• Equipment: Ensure the availability and functioning of all required equipment including:

- Oxygen source
- Functioning suction circuit
- Selection of appropriately sized ETTs with cuffs pretested for competence
- Laryngoscope with a selection of blades and a functioning light source
- Endotracheal stylet to form tube shape during intubation
- Self-inflating ventilation bag with attached oxygen feed
- Selection of face masks
- Selection of oral and nasal airways (Figure 27-5)
- Pulse oximeter to monitor patient oxygenation during procedure
- End-tidal CO_2 detector to determine correct tube placement following procedure

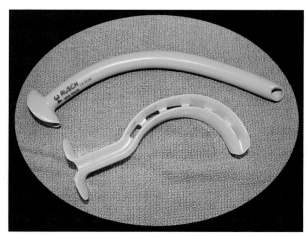

Figure 27-5. Nasal and oral airway.

- Mechanical ventilator: While a mechanical ventilator is not necessary for performance of the procedure, most patients will be placed on a mechanical ventilator immediately following intubation.

• Personnel

- Ensure the availability of skilled assistance during performance of procedure including respiratory therapist, nurse to monitor patient during performance of procedure and assist in procedure.

• Patient

- The patient should be preoxygenated prior to procedure (Figure 27-6), if possible, to minimize the possibility of desaturation during the procedure—this is typically done with a period of enriched oxygen breathing prior to endotracheal intubation.
- Positioning: The patient should be placed in the "sniffing" position with head flexed on torso, and neck extended, to optimize airway alignment (this can be done by putting the patient's head on a small pillow or by placing a towel roll behind the patient's neck). Elevate the head of the bed where possible.
- Ensure the availability of a free flowing intravenous catheter for medication administration.

—Procedure: The operator stands behind the patient's head prior to initiation of the procedure and prepares all equipment as above. While this is a nonsterile procedure, protective gloves should be worn to prevent direct contact with patient secretions.

• The operator typically preoxygenates the patient by holding a mask on the patient's face with the left hand and assisting or actively ventilating the patient with the self-inflating bag held in the right hand.

• When the patient is adequately oxygenated and/or sedated and paralyzed, the operator begins procedure.

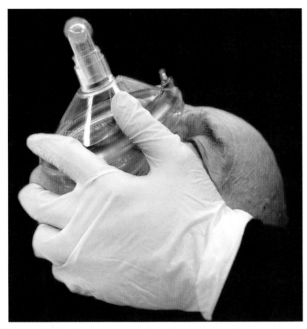

Figure 27-6. Preoxygenation (as viewed from the patient's left side) showing the hand position of the operator, who holds the mask in the left hand, gripping the mask with the thumb and index finger and the mandible with the remaining fingers.

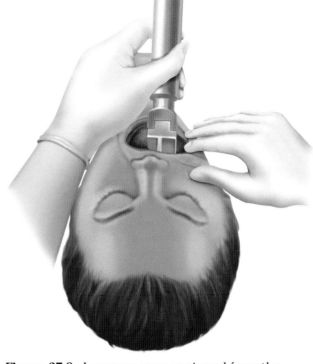

Figure 27-8. Laryngoscopy as viewed from the operator's vantage point.

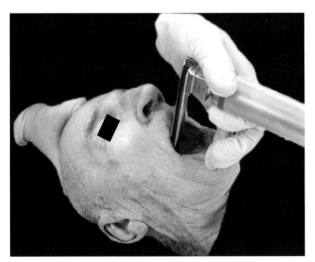

Figure 27-7. Insertion of the laryngoscope blade into the mouth.

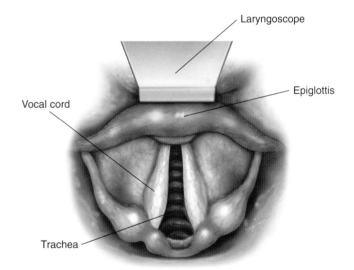

Figure 27-9. The vocal cords and surrounding anatomy.

- The laryngoscope is a left-handed instrument and should be in the operator's left hand in a "hammer grip" with the blade opened and the light on (Figure 27-7).
- The patient's mouth is opened with the thumb and index finger of the right hand and the blade of the laryngoscope is inserted in the patient's mouth (Figure 27-8).

- Pooled airway secretions may need to be suctioned at this point to enhance visualization of airway structures.
- The tip of the laryngoscope blade is advanced along the root of the tongue, lifting up and away from the operator until the epiglottis and vocal cords are exposed (Figure 27-9).

- At this point the oral, pharyngeal, and tracheal axes are aligned (Figure 27-10).
- The tip of the ETT is passed between the cords and advanced an additional several centimeters (Figures 27-11 to 27-12).
- The blade is withdrawn and the ETT cuff is inflated.
- End-tidal CO_2 verification is performed.

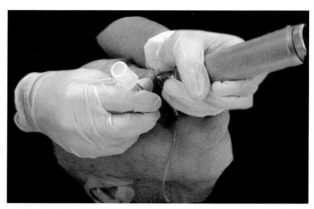

Figure 27-12. Advancement of the tube to correct position.

- The tube is secured using tape or one of a variety of tube securing devices.
- A chest film is performed to determine ETT tip position.

■ Nasal endotracheal intubation

—"Blind" nasal intubation differs from oral intubation primarily in the performance of the procedure—preparation is the same with the following exceptions.

- The patient should ideally be upright and the head placed in the "sniffing" position as above.
- If the patient is in the upright position, the operator stands to one side or the other of the patient (a right-handed operator will be facing the patient and on the patient's right so as to allow the dominant hand to be in the optimal position).
- If time permits, the nares should be compared for airflow (by occluding one and then the other and asking the patient to sniff).
- The more patent side should be prepared with a topical vasoconstrictor (ie, phenylephrine, oxymetolazone) and a topical anesthetic (ie, lidocaine).
- Sedation should be administered as appropriate.
- A well-lubricated ETT is then passed into the nostril and advanced into the nasopharynx, where breath sounds typically are audible.
- The ETT should be advanced to the point that breath sounds are loudest, which is typically just above the vocal cords.
- The tip of the tube is passed between the cords on inspiration (when the vocal cords are widely open), which often precipitates a cough (Figure 27-13).
- Breath sounds and air movement will continue to be audible through the ETT if it is correctly positioned in the trachea.

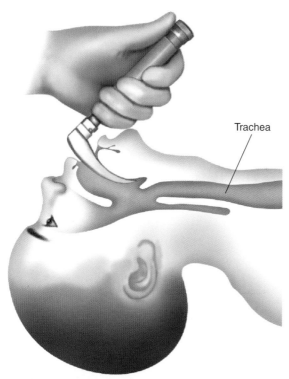

Trachea

Figure 27-10. Laryngoscopy, with the oral, pharyngeal, and tracheal axes aligned for optimal visualization.

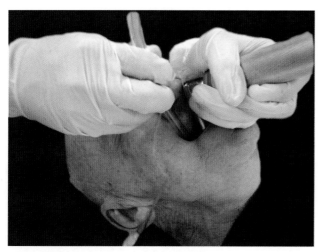

Figure 27-11. Insertion of the ETT.

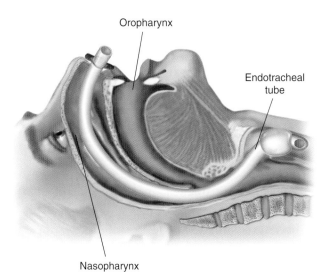

Figure 27-13. Tube position following nasotracheal intubation.

- If breath sounds and/or air movement is absent, the tube should be withdrawn and the head repositioned or the tube rotated a quarter of a turn clockwise or counterclockwise with each successive attempt.

- Successful endotracheal intubation should be confirmed with an end-tidal CO_2 detector.

- When successful intubation has been confirmed, the ETT cuff should be inflated and a chest film performed to verify tube position.

—Contraindications to nasotracheal intubation

- Coagulopathy (ie, therapeutic anticoagulation, thrombocytopenia)

- Inability to advance tube through either nostril due to anatomic obstruction (ie, nasal septal deviation).

- Precipitation of excessive nasal bleeding during procedure.

 Clinical Pearls and Pitfalls

▪ The Macintosh curved laryngoscope blade is used most commonly and is the easiest to use for inexperienced operators.

▪ In an emergency situation, a malleable stylet should be placed in the ETT prior to laryngoscopy and the tube should be bent so that the distal five centimeters are curved anteriorly (in the shape of a hockey stick).

▪ While several tubes should be available, a 7-mm internal diameter tube is typically used for adult females, while an 8-mm tube is used for adult males—both sizes are cuffed and will permit the passage of a bronchoscope.

▪ Ausculatation over the stomach during inspiration may reveal gurgling sounds and indicate esophageal intubation, which must be rectified *immediately*—some experts advocate leaving the misplaced tube in place with the cuff inflated while placing a new tube in the correct position to prevent regurgitation of stomach contents.

▪ Breath sounds may be inaudible and end-tidal CO_2 very difficult to detect in patients with severe bronchospasm; similarly end-tidal CO_2 may be very low or undetectable in patients with no circulation.

 Suggested Reading

Mort TC. Complications of emergency tracheal intubation: hemodynamic alterations; Part I. *J Intensive Care Med.* 2007;22:157–165.

Mort TC. Complications of emergency tracheal intubation: immediate airway-related consequences; Part II. *J Intensive Care Med.* 2007;22:208–215.

Percutaneous Airways

 Introduction

Percutaneous or surgical airways may be placed in patients in the intensive care unit for a variety of reasons including elective transition from an oral or nasal endotracheal tube to a chronic tracheostomy, or in emergency airway management (as described in Chapter 23). Alternative approaches include percutaneous tracheostomy and cricothyroidotomy.

 Definitions and Terms

- Larynx: The cartilaginous portion of the respiratory tract between the pharynx and the trachea, consisting of the cricoid cartilage, the thyroid cartilage and the arytenoids, the laryngeal muscles and the vocal cords (Figure 28-1)
- Cricothyroid membrane: A membrane between the thyroid cartilage and the cricoids cartilage

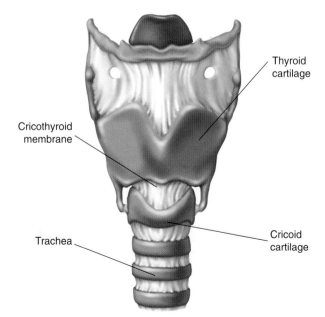

Figure 28-1. Laryngeal anatomy.

- Tracheostomy: Surgical creation of an opening from the skin into the trachea for the insertion of an artificial airway
- Cricothyroidotomy: Surgical creation of an opening between the skin and the trachea through the cricothyroid membrane
- Prolonged intubation: Oral or nasal intubation for a period exceeding several days—some evidence suggests that a percutaneous airway should be performed after 3 days of intuibation, whereas most would agree that it should be considered after 7 days

 Techniques

- Indications
  - Prolonged intubation
  - Airway obstruction (supraglottic)
  - Pulmonary toilet
  - Obstructive sleep apnea
  - Emergency airway management
- Contraindications
  - Infection or surgical incision close to proposed insertion site
  - Coagulopathy
  - Distorted neck anatomy
    - Prior surgery
    - Thyromegaly
    - Neck trauma
- Patient should be consented for procedure, the site prepped and draped, and universal protocol performed as per Section I.
  - Percutaneous tracheostomy
    - The patient should be positioned with the neck extended (Figure 28-2).
    - Sedation should be administered as needed.
    - If the procedure is elective, a bronchoscope should be inserted through the existing endotracheal tube.

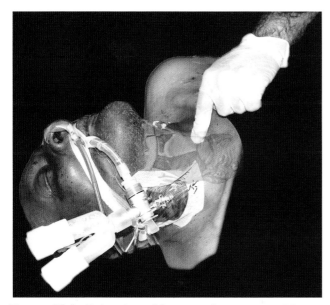

Figure 28-2. Palpation of laryngeal anatomy with underlying anatomy.

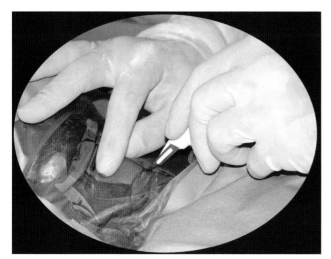

Figure 28-3. Skin incision with underlying anatomy.

- The tracheal rings should be palpated and the first and second rings identified.
- The skin overlying these rings should be anesthetized with local anesthetic and a transverse (or vertical) 1.5 to 2 cm incision made in the skin and blunt dissection performed down to the tracheal cartilage (Figure 28-3).
- Where feasible, a bronchoscope should be inserted into the trachea and to visualize insertion site, and the existing tracheal tube withdrawn (if applicable) far enough to permit simultaneous mechanical ventilation and endoscopic observation.

- A narrow gauge needle (18–22) is inserted into the trachea, and midline position visually verified by endoscopic observation (bronchoscopically)—alternatively a needle through catheter can be inserted and the needle withdrawn (Figure 28-4).

- A guidewire is inserted through the narrow gauge needle or catheter.

- A series of dilators are then inserted over the guidewire under endoscopic visualization (Figures 28-5 to 28-9).

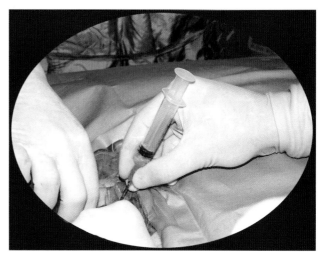

Figure 28-4. Needle insertion into trachea.

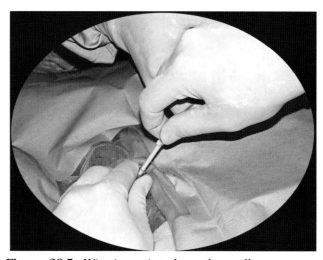

Figure 28-5. Wire insertion through needle.

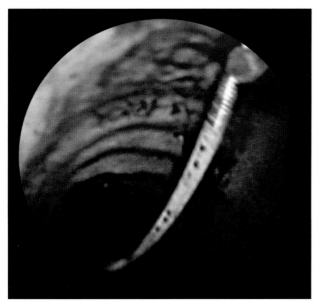

Figure 28-6. Bronchoscopic verification of correct wire position through anterior wall of trachea.

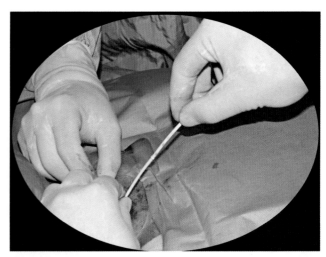

Figure 28-8. Passage of exchange "sleeve" over wire.

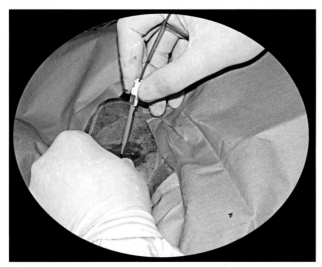

Figure 28-7. Passage of small dilator over wire.

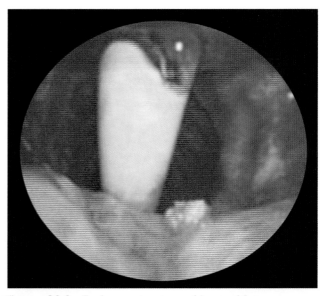

Figure 28-9. Endoscopic view of large dilator over wire and sleeve.

- The tracheostomy tube is inserted with the final dilator and the dilators and wire withdrawn (Figures 28-10 to 28-12).
- The tube is secured.
  - Cricothyroidotomy
- Performed exactly as the percutaneous tracheostomy, with the exception that the insertion site is through the cricothyroid membrane (Figure 28-13)

⚠ Clinical Pearls and Pitfalls

- Minor hemorrhage can be controlled with direct compression, whereas major hemorrhage warrants surgical exploration.
- Subcutaneous emphysema and potential pneumothorax can occur when the needle lacerates the trachea.
- The most common complication of these procedures is creation of a false passage.

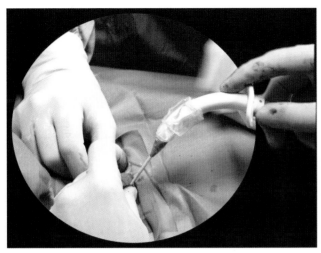

Figure 28-10. Passage of dilator and tracheostomy tube over sleeve.

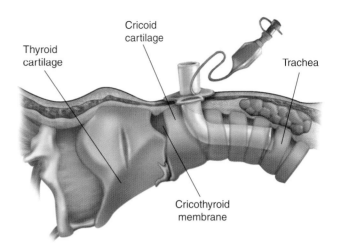

Figure 28-12. Graphic of tracheostomy tube and surrounding anatomy.

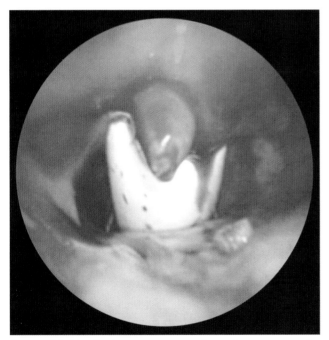

Figure 28-11. Endoscopic view of tracheostomy tube entering trachea.

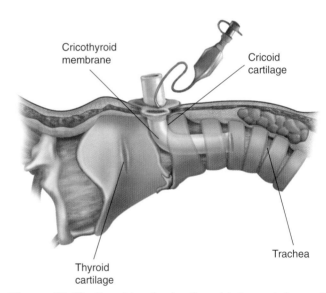

Figure 28-13. Graphic of cricothyroidotomy tube and surrounding anatomy (compare Figure 28-12).

- Tracheoarterial and tracheoesophageal fistulae are uncommon complications of the procedure.
- It is possible to lose control of the airway during the procedure if the endotracheal tube is withdrawn too far, prior to securing the percutaneous airway, in which case it is necessary to proceed quickly with completion of the surgical procedure or that procedure should be abandoned while oral intubation is performed.

 Suggested Reading

Walz MK, Peitgen K, Thurauf N, et al. Percutaneous dilatational tracheostomy—early results and long-term outcome of 326 critically ill patients. *J Intensive Care Med.* 1998;24:685–690.

Kahveci SF, Goren S, Kutlay O, et al. Bedside percutaneous tracheostomy experience with 72 critically ill patients. *Eur J Anaesthesiol.* 2000;17:688–691.

CHAPTER 29

Mechanical Ventilation

 Introduction

Mechanical ventilation is machine-supported respiratory support which may completely replace or assist the patient's spontaneous efforts. Mechanical ventilation is typically provided through an artificial airway, although mechanical ventilators may be used as an adjunct to noninvasive positive pressure ventilation. Negative pressure mechanical ventilation will not be discussed in this chapter, because its use is limited and a full discussion of all of the aspects of mechanical ventilation is beyond the scope of this chapter.

 Definitions and Terms

- Rate: The respiratory rate may be used to indicate machine or patient rate
  - Machine rate: The rate at which the ventilator delivers positive pressure ventilation
  - Patient rate: The patient's spontaneous respiratory rate
- Tidal volume (TV): The volume of each breath, and as with rate, this may be used to indicate mechanically delivered or patient TV
- Minute ventilation (V_E): The total volume of air breathed (whether spontaneous or mechanical) during 60 sec
- Fi_{O_2}: The inspired oxygen concentration
- Pressure: A variety of pressures are set and measured on a ventilator including:
  - Inspiratory pressure: Typically the pressure at which the ventilator delivers a breath, although it may also mean the pressure reached when the ventilator delivers a set volume of gas.
  - Trigger pressure: The negative pressure a patient mush achieve to initiate a ventilator supported breath.
  - Positive end-expiratory pressure (PEEP): The pressure the ventilator maintains during the expiratory phase of a breath.

- Sigh: A larger than normal breath delivered by the ventilator at preset intervals to expand collapsed alveoli
- Mode: One of a large number of ventilator settings that can be set to assist patient ventilation and thereby reduce work of breathing, including:
  - Control mode: The ventilator is set to deliver all of the ventilation.
  - Assist control (AC mode): The ventilator has asset minimum number of breaths and augments every patient respiratory effort with a preset TV.
  - Intermittent mandatory ventilation (typically synchronized or SIMV): The ventilator supports a preset number of breaths with a preset TV, and the patient may generate additional spontaneous TV.
  - Pressure support: Every patient effort is supported with positive pressure at a preset level—TVs may vary from supported breath to supported breath.
  - High frequency ventilation: One of a variety of approaches to ventilatory support wherein mechanical respiratory rate is supranormal—usually with smaller than normal TVs.

 Techniques

- There are a variety of indications for mechanical ventilation ranging from short term (ie, perioperative) to chronic (ie, chronic respiratory failure).
  - Intraoperative
  - Postrespiratory or cardiac arrest
  - Chronic obstructive pulmonary disease (COPD) exacerbation
  - Asthma
  - Acute respiratory failure
  - Neurologic failure
  - Cardiogenic shock/pulmonary edema
- Contraindications to mechanical ventilation.
  - Presence of an advanced directive precluding its application

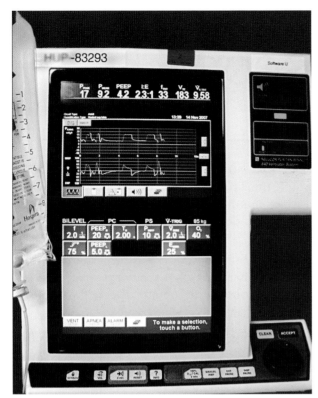

Figure 29-1. Mechanical ventilator showing respiratory waveforms.

- The ventilator (Figure 29-1) is connected to the artificial airway using a standard connector.
- Initial Fi_{O_2}, rate, and mode are selected depending on the patient's clinical status.
- Ventilator alarms should be set to recognize patient disconnection, high respiratory rate, low TV, and/or minute ventilation.
- Provisions should be made to ensure humidification of inspired gases using either an in-line humidifier or artificial nose.
- The head of the bed should be maintained at 45°, and the oropharynx and endotracheal tube suctioned frequently to minimize the likelihood of ventilator associated pneumonia.
- The patient should be reassessed frequently to optimize the effectiveness of MV, and to evaluate whether there is an ongoing requirement for MV.
- MV should be discontinued as soon as patient status permits.

 ## Clinical Pearls and Pitfalls

- Noninvasive positive pressure ventilation may be adequate as an alternative to MV in certain patient populations.
- Institutional consensus protocols for the weaning of MV in acute and chronically ventilated populations as well as spontaneous breathing trials may shorten the duration of mechanical ventilation.
- New evidence suggests that reduced TVs in certain patient populations (ie, acute respiratory distress syndrome [ARDS]) are associated with improved outcome.
- Patients undergoing positive pressure ventilation are at increased risk from pneumothorax, and that diagnosis should be considered in any patient with acute hemodynamic deterioration on a ventilator.
- Similarly, patients are at increased risk for auto-PEEP (ie, air-trapping) and this diagnosis should be considered in patients with obstructive airways disease (ie, COPD and asthma) and acute hemodynamic compromise.

 ## Suggested Reading

http://www.ccmtutorials.com/rs/mv/index.htm

Hess DR. Mechanical ventilation strategies: What's new and what's worth keeping? *Respir Care*. 2002;47: 1007–1017.

Tobin MJ. *Principles and Practice of Mechanical Ventilation*. 2nd ed. New York: McGraw-Hill; 2006.

CHAPTER 30

Bronchoscopy

 Introduction

Bronchoscopy is frequently performed both as a diagnostic and therapeutic maneuver in the intensive care unit (ICU), wherein a flexible endoscope is threaded into the airways. The bronchoscope has a fiberoptic light source and suction channels as well as cables allowing the tip of the device to be flexed and retroflexed in one plane (Figure 30-1).

 Definitions and Terms

- Fiberoptic bronchoscope (FOB): Commonly used in the ICU.
- Rigid bronchoscope: Inflexible variant bronchoscope not typically used in the ICU.

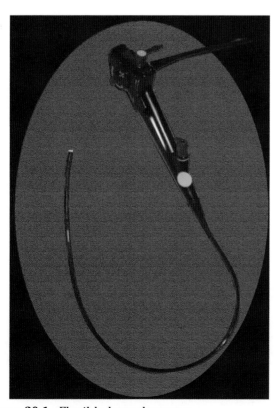

Figure 30-1. Flexible bronchoscope.

- Fiberoptic intubation: Endotracheal intubation in which the bronchoscope is advanced through the nose or mouth and into the proximal trachea, after which an endotracheal tube is threaded over it into the airway.
- Diagnostic bronchoscopy: May be performed to evaluate the character of the airways (ie, for edema, bleeding source), to obtain selected pathological specimens (ie, cultures, or tissue).
- Therapeutic bronchoscopy: May be performed to remove secretions, clots, or foreign bodies from the airways.

 Techniques

- Prior to performance of bronchoscopy, consent and the universal protocol should be performed as in Section I.
- The operator should determine the approach to bronchoscopy.
  - Awake-sedated bronchoscopy: This approach may be selected for patients in whom there is no need for an endotracheal tube and involves topical anesthesia of the proximal airway as well as sedation.
  - Endotracheal: This approach is more common in patients in the ICU in whom bronchoscopy is performed through an existing artificial airway (ie, endotracheal tube or tracheostomy) as in Figure 30-2.
- The operator should be familiar with proximal airway anatomy (Figure 30-3).
- The bronchoscope can be advanced and withdrawn and the tip can be flexed with a thumb control to navigate the airways (Figure 30-4)—the index finger is used to control suction.
- Airway bifurcations should be identified and may be off-axis depending on the operator's location relative to the patient and the rotation of the tip of the bronchoscope relative to the hand control (Figures 30-5 to 30-6).

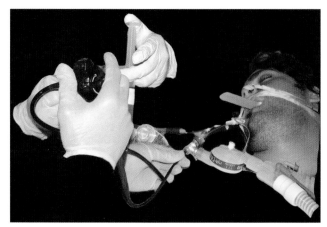

Figure 30-2. Bronchoscopy through an endotracheal tube in an intubated patient.

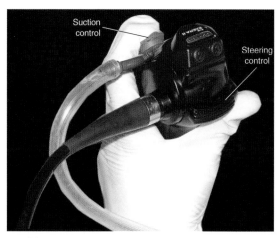

Figure 30-4. The hand controls of a flexible bronchoscope.

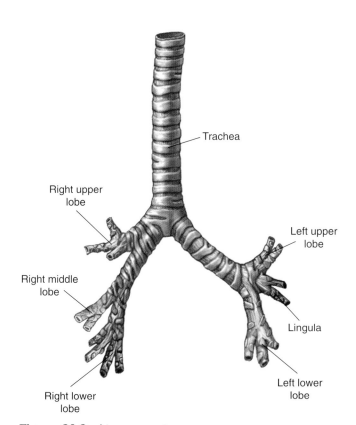

Figure 30-3. Airway anatomy.

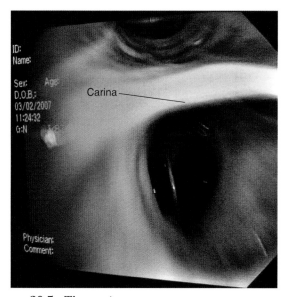

Figure 30-5. The carina.

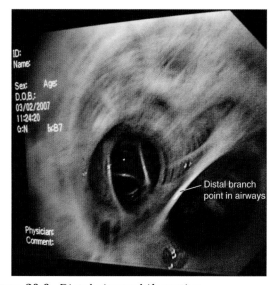

Figure 30-6. Distal airway bifurcation.

- Secretions (Figure 30-7), blood, pus, or foreign bodies may be identified in the airway and should be removed to prevent atelectasis.
- Suctioned material can be captured from the suction line and sent for culture or pathologic identification (Figure 30-8).

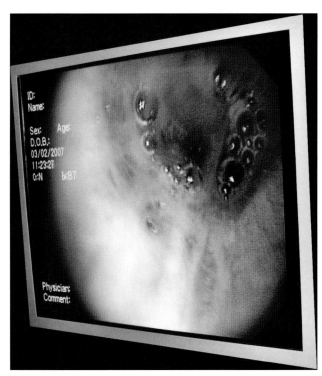

Figure 30-7. Secretions occluding an airway.

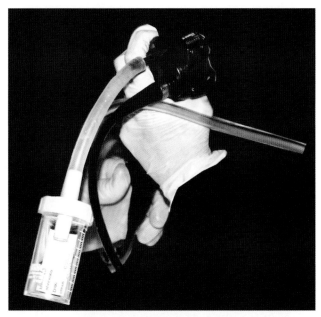

Figure 30-8. Trap to acquire suctioned secretions from the bronchoscopic suction channel.

 Clinical Pearls and Pitfalls

- Preparation is essential to efficient and safe performance of bronchoscopy—prior to the procedure, the scope's focus should be adjusted, lenses defogged, and the scope shaft lubricated for smooth passage through the artificial airway.
- Attachment of the bronchoscope to a video monitor may facilitate performance of the procedure by allowing the operator to work in a head-up position.
- The patient should be placed on high inspired Fi_{O_2} and sedated during the procedure so as to prevent coughing and oxygen desaturation.
- The operator should have appropriate assistance during the procedure (ie, nursing and respiratory therapy)—the patient's respiratory and vital signs should be monitored throughout.
- Saline lavage and irrigation may facilitate removal of thick secretions from the airways.

 Suggested Reading

Dakin J, Griffiths M. The pulmonary physician in critical care 1: pulmonary investigations for acute respiratory failure. *Thorax.* 2002;57:79–85.

CHAPTER 31

Thoracentesis

 ## Introduction

Thoracentesis is a procedure by which fluid is removed from either hemithorax through a needle or small catheter inserted for that purpose, and may be a diagnostic or therapeutic procedure.

 ## Definitions and Terms

- Pleural tap: Typically used to describe a diagnostic thoracentesis
- Transudate: Pleural fluid where pathologic analysis of the fluid shows little protein and few cells—consistent with several primary etiologies
  —Congestive heart failure
  —Hypoalbuminemia
  —Nephritic syndrome
  —Cirrhosis
  —Atelectasis or trapped lung
- Exudate: Pleural fluid with protein and or cells
  —Pleural or pulmonary malignancy
  —Hemorrhage
  —Connective tissue disease
  —Pulmonary embolism
  —Lymphatic disease

 ## Techniques

- There are many indications for thoracentesis that can generally be categorized under one of two headings:
  —Diagnostic: Evaluation of pleural fluid to diagnose primary disease process
  —Therapeutic: Done to drain fluid to improve respiratory status of the patient
- Contraindications.
  —Bleeding diathesis (ie, low platelets, abnormal coagulation parameters)
  —Small effusion with significant risk of injury to the lung during performance of the procedure
  —Bullous disease on the side of the effusion
  —Positive pressure ventilation (relative)
- The location of the effusion should be identified radiographically (ie, chest x-ray, CT scan, or ultrasound).
- Prior to procedure, the patient should be consented, prepped, and the universal protocol should be performed as per Section I.
- The patient is typically positioned in an upright position allowing fluid to settle at the bottom of the hemithorax, and percussion may be used to identify the interface between lung and fluid (Figure 31-1).
- The site is marked and local anesthetic infiltrated down to the rib (Figure 31-2).
- A needle is introduced into the pleural space and fluid withdrawal confirmed (Figure 31-3).
- A catheter is then inserted into the effusion using one of a variety of techniques, including catheter-through-needle, catheter-over-needle, and Seldinger exchange (Figure 31-4).

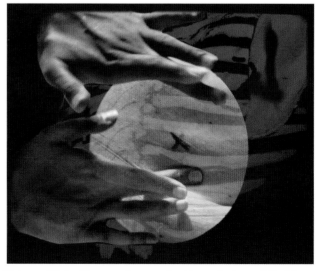

Figure 31-1. Percussive evaluation of pleural fluid meniscus.

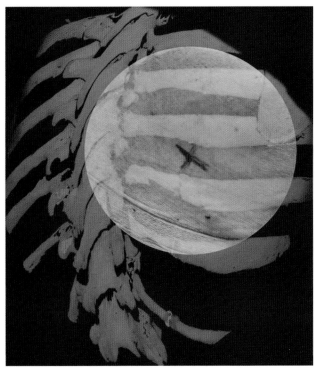

Figure 31-2. Site marked for needle insertion.

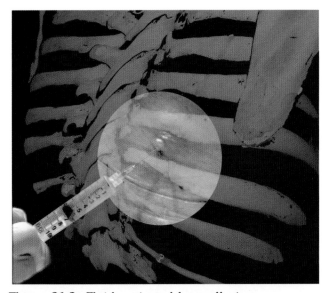

Figure 31-3. Fluid aspirated from effusion.

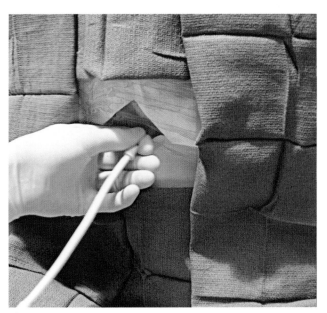

Figure 31-4. Catheter threaded into chest cavity.

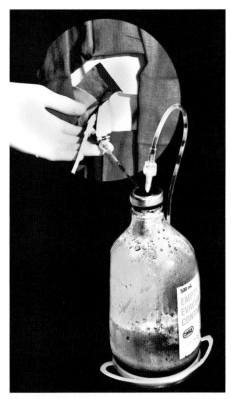

Figure 31-5. Pleural fluid drained into vacuum bottle.

- The fluid is then drained into a vacuum bottle (Figure 31-5) or drainage bag.
- The fluid is then sent off for appropriate diagnostic studies.

 Clinical Pearls and Pitfalls

- The drainage catheter may stop draining if the tip sucks up against lung or pleura, in which case the patient can be repositioned to move the effusion around in the thorax.

- Drainage may significantly less than the apparent size of the effusion when fluid is loculated.

- Pneumothorax can result from the procedure if the lung is injured or if air is entrained into the chest during a spontaneous negative-pressure inspiration.

- Removal of greater than 1 L of fluid from a single hemithorax at a single setting can be associated with reexpansion pulmonary edema.

 ## Suggested Reading

Light RW. Pleural effusion. *N Engl J Med.* 2002;346: 1971–1977.

Thomsen TW, DeLaPena J, Setnik GS. Thoracentesis. *N Engl J Med.* 2006;355:e16.

CHAPTER 32

Tube Thoracostomy

 Introduction

Tube thoracostomy, commonly known as chest tube placement, is the insertion of a tube into the pleural space typically to drain air or fluid, although the procedure may be performed for pleurodesis or lysis of adhesions in the pleural space.

 Definitions and Terms

- Pneumothorax: Accumulation of air in the pleural space
- Pleural effusion: Accumulation of fluid in the pleural space
- Pleurodesis: Medical treatment for refractory pleural effusion (often malignant) or pneumothorax in which a chemical is instilled into the pleural space to adhere the pleural and pulmonary surfaces to one another

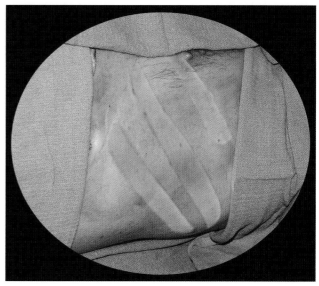

Figure 32-1. Draped and prepped incision site in med-axillary line.

 Techniques

- There are a variety of indications for tube thoracostomy.
  - Aspiration of air from a pneumothorax or with bronchopleural fistula
  - Therapeutic drainage of serous, infected, or malignant fluid from the chest
  - Postoperative drainage of the chest following thoracic or cardiac surgery
  - Trauma
- Contraindications.
  - Coagulopathy
  - Pleural adhesions
- The patient should be consented, prepped, and the universal protocol performed as in Section I.
- The patient is typically positioned on supine with the arm abducted over the head (Figure 32-1) for tube insertion in the mid-axillary line, although alternative positions may be appropriate.
- Local anesthesia is instilled into the area of insertion (Figure 32-2).

- A small 2-cm incision is made.
- The appropriate tube is inserted depending on the pathology.
  - Pneumothorax—small bore tube (ie, 8-18 French)
  - Fluid drainage—large bore tube (ie, 18 and above French)

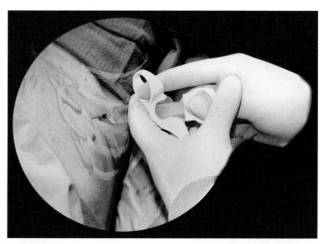

Figure 32-2. Skin infiltration with local anesthetic.

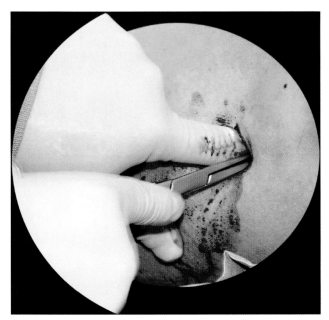

Figure 32-3. Blunt finger dissection.

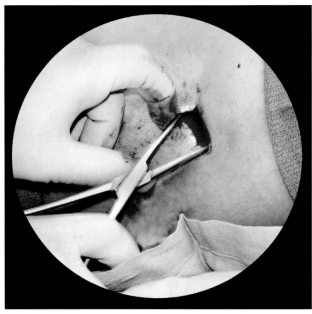

Figure 32-5. Widening of pleural opening with hemostat.

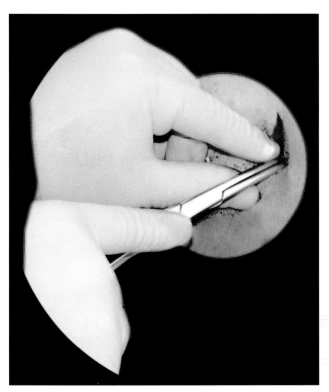

Figure 32-4. Hemostat dissection.

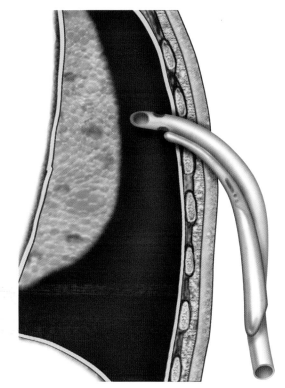

Figure 32-6. Tube guided into pleural space with hemostat.

- Small tubes can be inserted using Seldinger technique.
- Larger tubes are inserted using blunt dissection (Figures 32-3 to 32-5).
- If blunt dissection is used, a hemostat is used to guide the tube into the thoracic cavity (Figure 32-6).

- The tube should be directed appropriately depending on the nature of the pathology, that is, cephalad for a pneumothorax (Figure 32-7) or posteriorly and inferiorly for an effusion.

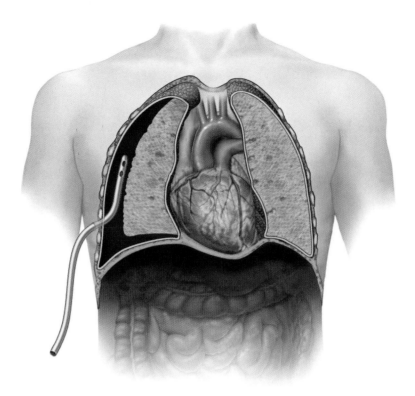

Figure 32-7. Tube threaded apically in patient with pneumothorax.

- The chest tube should be attached to a drainage system and monitored for ongoing fluid drainage and air leak.
- A chest x-ray should be performed following the procedure to ascertain tube position (Figure 32-8).

! Clinical Pearls and Pitfalls

- A finger should be inserted into the incision to ensure that there is a free space surrounding the lung into which the tube may be placed.

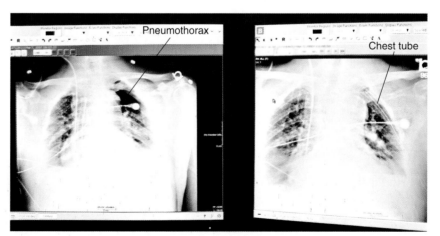

Figure 32-8. Before and after chest x-rays in patient with pneumothorax.

- Complications of tube placement include lung laceration, misplacement relative to the pathology, that is, effusion or air not drained because of tube position in fissure, under diaphragm or in subcutaneous tissue

- The tube may become occluded, kinked, or dislodged.

- The tube should be withdrawn during patient exhalation and the site immediately sealed with petrolatum gauze to prevent pneumothorax.

 ## Suggested Reading

Dev SP, Nascimiento B, Simone C, Chien V. Chest-tube insertion. *N Engl J Med*. 2007;357:e15.

Laws D, Neville E, Duffy J. BTS guidelines for the insertion of a chest drain. *Thorax*. 2003;58(suppl 2): ii53–ii59.

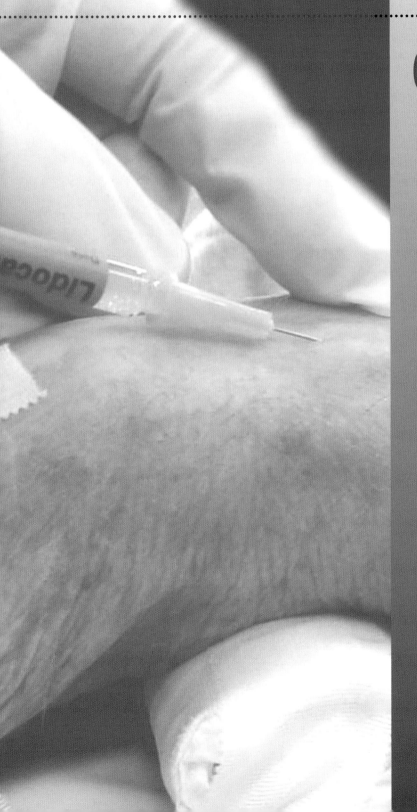

Cardiovascular Procedures

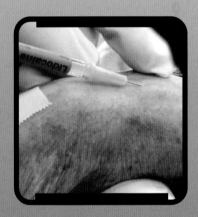

CHAPTER 33

Electrocardiography

 Introduction

Electrocardiography (ECG) is a standard intensive care unit monitoring modality both in the continuous and twelve lead formats. It is used both for the detection of cardiac ischemia and arrhythmias.

 Definitions and Terms

- ECG waves (Figure 33-1)
  - P wave—initial electrocardiographic deflection from the baseline in a cardiac contraction—corresponds to the electrical activation of the atria following sinoatrial node depolarization
  - PR interval—corresponds to the period of atrial conduction through the atrioventricular node
  - QRS complex—corresponds to electrical activation of the ventricles
  - ST segment—segment connecting the QRS complex to the T wave, and may indicate coronary ischemia (if depressed below baseline) or myocardial infarction (if elevated above baseline)
  - T wave—corresponds to repolarization of the ventricles
- ECG lead—used to mean both the electrical wire connecting the patient to the ECG machine, and one of the axes of cardiac electrical conduction commonly evaluated by ECG.
  - Limb leads show conduction between any two of the three limbs comprising Einthoven's triangle (right arm, left arm, left leg) as shown in Figure 33-2. Green is traditionally used as a ground lead.
  - Lead vector—shows the direction of conduction between the negative and positive terminals of a given lead as shown in 12-lead ECG in Figure 33-3
    - Limb leads

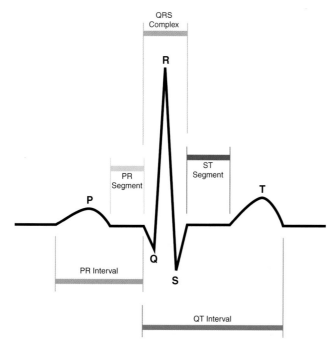

Figure 33-1. Standard electrical waves, waveforms and intervals on an ECG trace for a single heartbeat.

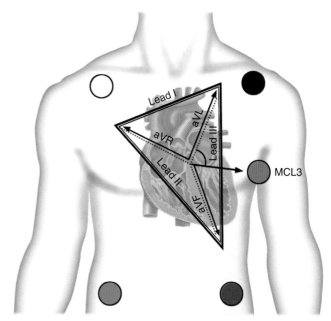

Figure 33-2. Einthoven's triangle, named after one of the inventors of the ECG, showing the various leads of the standard ECG.

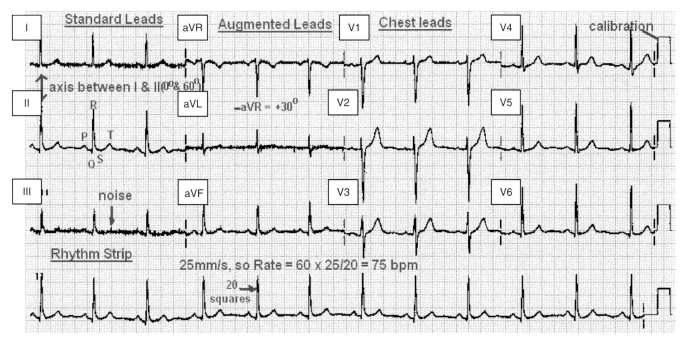

Figure 33-3. Standard 12-lead ECG showing each of the leads and the typical direction of conduction (positive or negative) between the two terminals of the lead.

- Lead I shows the axis of conduction from the right arm (white lead) to the left arm (black lead), with an upward deflection indicating conduction from right to left.

- Lead II shows the axis of conduction from the right arm toward the left leg (red lead).

- Lead III shows the axis of conduction from the left shoulder toward the left leg.

—Augmented limb leads show the axis of conduction from an imaginary central location (comprised of the center point between the three reference limbs) toward those limbs.

- aVR shows electrical conduction from the central lead toward the right arm.

- aVL shows conduction from the central lead to the left arm.

- aVF shows conduction from the central lead to the left leg (or foot).

- Precordial leads show conduction from the imaginary central point toward various locations on the chest wall (Figure 33-4).

- V_1 is placed in the fourth intercostals space on the right side of the sternum.

- V_2 is placed in the fourth intercostals space to the left of the sternum.

- V_3 is placed midway between leads V_2 and V_4.

- V_4 is placed in the fifth intercostals space in the midclavicular line.

- V_5 is placed next to V_4 but in the anterior axillary line.

- V_6 is placed next to V_5 but in the midaxillary line.

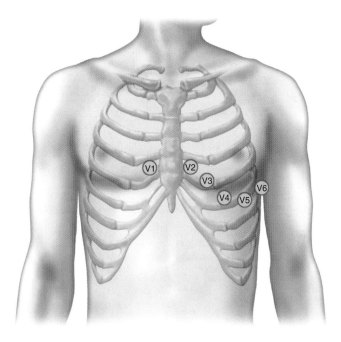

Figure 33-4. The precordial leads and their placement on the chest.

- Modified chest leads closely approximate true precordial leads, so MCL1 (modified chest lead 1) approximates V_1 etc.
  - Ground lead—the green lead often placed by convention of the right leg, but can be anywhere on the body and used to limit electrical noise

 ## Techniques

- A 12-lead ECG (leads I, II, III, aVR, aVL, aVF, V_1, V_2, V_3, V_4, V_5, V_6) may be acquired on admission to the intensive care unit, or at any time during and ICU stay to evaluate for changes relative to prior ECGs, assess for ischemia or any of a variety of electrolyte disturbances or other cardiac problems that may be apparent from a twelve lead.

- In practice, lead placement may vary depending on wound dressing and patient anatomy (Figure 33-5).

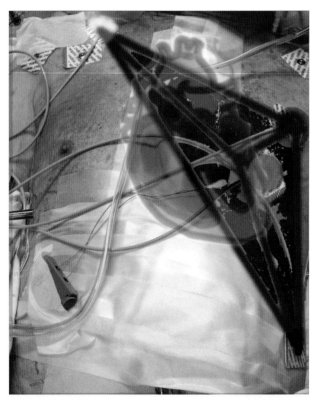

Figure 33-5. The placement of leads on an actual patient with wound dressings and consequently altered lead placement.

- Patients are usually monitored with one or two continuous ECG leads during ICU stay.
  - Lead II is often selected because it shows both the P wave and QRS complexes well, and can therefore be used to evaluate conduction abnormalities between the atria and ventricles (ie, atrial fibrillation).
  - Lead V_5 is often selected because it shows left ventricular ischemic problems most effectively.
- Many ICUs are equipped with automated arrhythmia detection systems which alarm when various critical arrhythmias are detected, but may be susceptible to artifact.

 ## Clinical Pearls and Pitfalls

- Continuous electrocardiographic traces may appear to show findings such as ST-segment elevation which are not confirmed on a standard twelve lead, which should always be performed when electrocardiographic anomalies are detected.

- Poor adherence of ECG leads to the skin is a major source of artifact, and leads should be clean, dry, and attached to the patient with conducting gel.

- ECG interpretation is a complicated and a full discussion of all possible findings would fill a book.

- Automated ECG interpretations are increasingly accurate, but an expert interpretation is warranted when automated reading is suspect or inconsistent with clinical findings.

 ## Suggested Reading

Galen S. Wagner. *Marriott's Practical Electrocardiography, 11th Edition* Philadelphia. Lippincott Williams and Wilkins; 2007.

http://www.americanheart.org/presenter.jhtml?identifier=3004613

CHAPTER 34

Catheter Insertion

 Introduction

Intravascular devices and catheters can be inserted in the intensive care unit (ICU) for a variety of purposes, including fluid and drug administration, pressure monitoring, pacemaking, or cardiac augmentation. Several techniques can be used to obtain access to and cannulate the vessel. Parenthetically, these same techniques can be used for other procedures such as thoracentesis or paracentesis.

 Definitions and Terms

- Needle through catheter: Large bore needle inserted into vessel and smaller bore catheter threaded through needle into vessel
- Catheter over needle: smaller bore needle inserted into vessel and large bore catheter threaded over needle into vessel
- Seldinger technique: Small bore needle inserted into vessel, wire passed through needle into vessel, needle removed, catheter threaded over wire into vessel, wire removed
- Modified Seldinger technique: Small bore needle inserted into vessel, wire passed through needle into vessel, needle removed, dilator/sheath passed over wire into vessel, wire and dilator removed, catheter threaded through sheath into vessel, sheath removed

 Techniques

- Vessel identification
  - Anatomy: Some vessels are identified primarily through anatomic landmarks.
    - Internal jugular: Typically cannulated at the apex of the triangle formed by the sternal and clavicular portions of the sternocleidomastoid muscle and the clavicle, wherein the needle is inserted at this location and aimed toward the ipsilateral nipple

    - Subclavian vein: Typically passes under the clavicle in the midclavicular line, and the needle is inserted so as to pass under the clavicle at this point aiming toward the sterna notch
  - Pulses: Vessel location may be indicated by arterial pulse.
  - The internal jugular vein is typically adjacent and lateral to the internal carotid artery.
  - The femoral vein is medial to the femoral artery in the groin.
  - Ultrasound: Increasingly portable, high fidelity ultrasound devices are available at the bedside to guide vascular cannulation.
- Vessel cannulation
  - Direct cannulation: The needle is inserted into the vessel and a catheter is threaded directly over it into the vessel (Figure 34-1).
  - Transfixion: The needle is passed through both the front and back walls of the vessel and withdrawn until there is free blood flow, at which point the cannula is threaded off of the needle into the vessel (Figure 34-2).
  - Seldinger variants: The vessel is cannulated with a needle or catheter as above, and a wire is passed into the vessel over which dilators or catheters can readily be exchanged while access to the vessel is maintained with the wire (Figure 34-3).

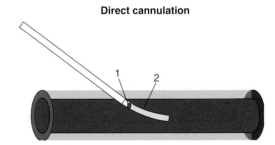

Direct cannulation

Figure 34-1. Direct cannulation, wherein (1) the vessel is cannulated and the (2) the catheter is threaded over the needle.

Transfixion

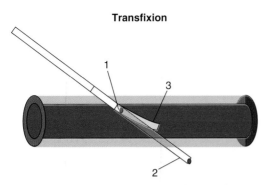

Figure 34-2. Transfixion, in which (1) the front and (2) the back walls of the vessel are transfixed after which the needle is withdrawn until there is free blood flow, at which point (3) the catheter is threaded into the vessel over the needle.

Seldinger technique

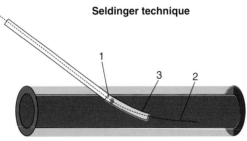

Figure 34-3. One of the Seldinger variants, in (1) which the vessel is cannulated with a catheter over needle technique, (2) the catheter is threaded over the needle into the vessel, and (3) a wire is threaded into the vessel through the catheter to act as an exchange device for larger catheters.

Clinical Pearls and Pitfalls

- When cannulating a vessel using the direct approach, the needle tip may be lodged in the vessel of interest while the catheter is still outside of the vessel in the subcutaneous tissue—attempts to thread the catheter at this point may push the vessel wall away from the catheter dislodging the needle from the vessel.

- A syringe should be attached to the needle during all major vascular cannulation attempts both as a diagnostic tool and to avoid air entrainment when cannulating a major vein.

- A vein may be compressed during cannulation, and it may therefore be unapparent to the operator when the needle enters the vessel—this problem can be avoided by alternating small needle advances into the tissue with syringe aspiration.

- The cannulation site should be below the level of the heart when cannulating major veins in a spontaneously ventilating patient who may entrain air into the vessel during negative pressure inspiration with resulting air embolism.

Suggested Reading

Higgs ZC, Macafee DA, Braithwaite BD, Maxwell-Armstrong CA. The Seldinger technique: 50 years on. *Lancet.* 2005;366:1407–1409.

CHAPTER 35

Arterial Line Cannulation

 Introduction

Arterial catheterization is a common procedure in medical and surgical intensive care units (ICUs). Arterial catheters are used for blood pressure monitoring in hemodynamically unstable patients and frequent arterial sampling in mechanically ventilated patients; the arterial line may also have been placed in the operating room prior to ICU arrival in perioperative patients.

 Definitions and Terms

- Arterial cannulation or catheterization: Insertion of a catheter into an artery for the purposes of continuous blood pressure transduction or arterial blood sampling
- Transducer: An electronic device that converts blood pressure into an electrical signal translated by a physiologic monitor into a numeric value—requires a reference, atmospheric value (ie, zeroing)

 Techniques

- Indications for arterial line placement.
  - Need for continuous (real-time) blood pressure monitoring
  - Hemodynamic instability necessitating the use and titration of inotropes or vasopressors
  - Need for reliable access to the arterial circulation for measurement of arterial oxygenation, arterial carbon dioxide, and/or frequent blood sampling
- Contraindications.
  - Compromised flow distal to cannulation site precludes cannulation on that side
  - Injury distal to cannulation site
  - Infection in the skin or subcutaneous tissues around cannulation site (ie, cellulitis)
  - Systemic anticoagulation (relative)
- Prior to procedure, obtain patient consent, prep and drape, and perform universal protocol as described in Section I.

- Identify cannulation site based on patient anatomy and clinical situation (Figure 35-1 and Table 35-1).
- Preparation.
  - Skin: The CDC recommends preparation of the cannulation site with a 2% aqueous chlorhexidine-gluconate solution, which has been associated with lower blood stream infection rates than povidine-iodine or alcohol-based preparations.

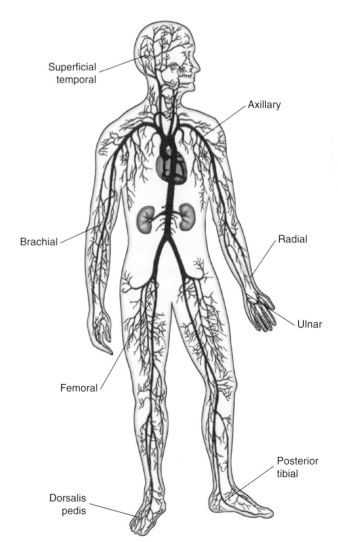

Figure 35-1. Arteries of the body with specific arterial cannulation sites.

Table 35-1. Table showing attributes of various cannulation sites.

Arterial Cannulation Sites

Site	Ease of cannulation	Advantages	Disadvantages
Radial	Easy, superficial	Superficial, distal, readily secured	Few
Femoral	Easy, superficial	Readily palpated, accurately reflects blood pressure	Infectious risk, requires the patient to remain recumbent
Brachial	Superficial, but the vessel can be mobile	Acceptable alternative to radial, readily secured (requires longer catheter)	Anatomic end-artery, potential for median nerve injury
Axillary	Difficult, particularly in obese or muscular patients	Accurate waveforms	Infectious risk, difficult to secure
Ulnar	Relatively easy, but deeper than radial	Similar to radial (but should not be attempted after failed radial attempts on same side)	
Dorsalis pedis	Easy, superficial	Superficial, distal, readily secured	
Posterior tibial	Relativelyeasy	Distal	
Temporal	Tortuous	None	Cosmetically awkward, should be regarded as site of last resort

The skin and tissue around the artery should be infiltrated with 1% lidocaine solution, except in patients with a known allergy to lidocaine, in whom alternative local anesthetics can be used.

—Hygiene: The operator should observe proper hand hygiene by washing hands with antiseptic soap, gel, or foam prior to palpation of the cannulation site or insertion, replacement, manipulation, or dressing of the catheter or site.

—Equipment: The cannula used for intra-arterial cannulation is typically a polyurethane or polyethylene catheter. The catheter size and length is typically determined by the size and depth of the artery of interest. Shorter, smaller catheters (ie, 20–22 gauge, 25–50 mm) are typically used when cannulating arteries in the hands and feet; whereas longer and thicker catheters (ie, 14–20 gauge, 15–20 cm) are used for larger vessels. The catheter should be connected to a disposable transducer using noncompliant tubing, which transmits the arterial waveform to the transducer with optimal fidelity.

—Operator: The CDC recommends that the operator wear sterile gloves for the placement of arterial catheters.

▪Methods (see Chapter 34 on vessel cannulation).

—Direct cannulation (Figures 35-2 to 35-6)

—Transfixion

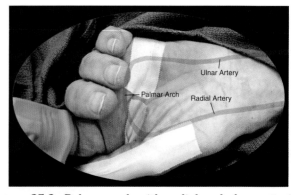

Figure 35-2. Palmar arch with radial and ulnar arteries.

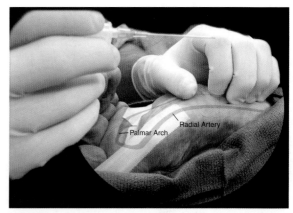

Figure 35-3. Palpation of pulse prior to cannulation of vessel.

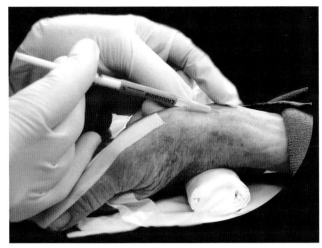

Figure 35-4. Infiltration of cannulation site with local anesthetic.

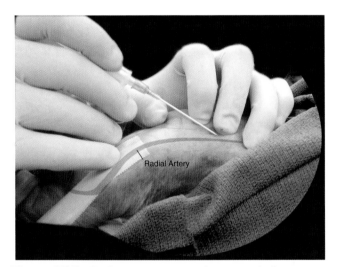

Figure 35-5. Catheter insertion during radial cannulation.

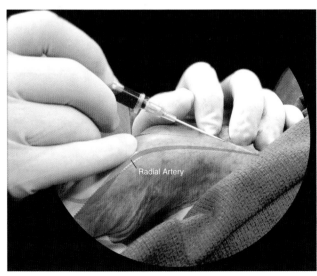

Figure 35-6. Arterial back-bleeding into cannula.

—Seldinger technique

—Ultrasound guided

—Cut down

- Monitoring: After placement, the catheter is attached to a pressure transducer zeroed to the level of the right atrium with high-pressure tubing and tracked on a bedside physiologic monitor. A continuous flush solution, with or without heparin, is used to maintain catheter patency.

- Monitor arterial wave trace for normal waveform, systolic and diastolic pressures (Figure 35-7).

- Complications.

  —Arterial vasospasm: Typically transient, less likely when perivascular area infiltrated with local anesthetic prior to cannulation

  —Infection: Infectious risk typically lower with arterial cannulas than venous catheters due to the flow velocity in the vessel

  —Dissection: More likely with cannulation of larger vessels such as femoral artery

  —Transection: More likely when larger needles are used to cannulate relatively smaller vessels such as radial artery

  —Thrombosis: More likely in patients with low-flow states, when catheter cross section is large relative to the size of the vessel

  —Embolization: Both clot and air can be embolized distally with catheter flushing

  —Hematoma: More likely in the presence of systemic anticoagulation, and after multiple cannulation attempts

  —Aneurysm formation: Unusual and more likely in patients with very calcified arteries

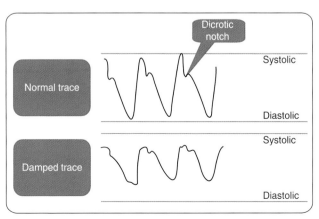

Figure 35-7. Normal and damped arterial waveforms.

Clinical Pearls and Pitfalls

- The Allen's test, historically used to determine the patency of the palmar arch, has been shown to be neither sufficiently sensitive nor specific to make it appropriate for clinical use.

- Fully extend the joint adjacent to the artery prior to cannulation to "fix" the vessel under tension, thereby minimizing vessel movement while cannulating. For example, the wrist is commonly dorsiflexed over a roll and secured to a board prior to cannulation (see Figure 35-4) to fix the radial artery along its long axis.

Suggested Reading

Russell JA, Joel M, Hudson RJ, Mangano DT, Schlobohm RM. Prospective evaluation of radial and femoral artery catheterization sites in critically ill adults. *Crit Care Med.* 1983;11:936–939.

CHAPTER 36

Central Venous Catheterization

 Introduction

Central veins are routinely cannulated in the intensive care unit (ICU) for pressure monitoring, drug administration and access to large vessels for procedures such as hemodialysis or administration of parenteral nutrition.

 Definitions and Terms

- Central venous catheter (CVC): Typically a catheter whose tip lies within the thorax, although a femoral venous catheter may be considered a CVC
- Central venous pressure: The pressure measured at the tip of a CVC
- Multilumen CVC: CVC with multiple separate channels with orifices lying at varying points along the catheter—each lumen can be treated as a separate fluid path
- Antibiotic impregnated catheter: A CVC impregnated with chlorhexidine, silver sulfadiazine, minocycline, and/or rifampin designed to decrease the rate of CVC associated infections
- Internal jugular (IJ)
- Subclavian vein (SCV)

 Techniques

- Indications for central line placement.
  - Central venous pressure monitoring
  - Administration of vesicant drugs that cause phlebitis or pain in peripheral, slow flowing veins
  - Alternative access when peripheral veins are unavailable due to dehydration, hemorrhage, or prior intravenous access with scarring
  - Parenteral nutrition

- Contraindications.
  - Coagulopathy
  - Skin infection
  - Contralateral carotid disease, where IJ cannulation may result in injury to remaining (ipsilateral) carotid
  - Subclavian cannulation when contralateral lung is diseased or absent, and ipsilateral pneumothorax puts patient at relatively increased risk
- Prior to procedure, obtain patient consent, prep and drape, and perform universal protocol as described in Section I.
- Identify cannulation site based on patient anatomy and clinical situation (Figure 36-1 and Table 36-1).
- Preparation.
  - Skin: The CDC recommends preparation of the cannulation site with a 2% aqueous chlorhexidine-gluconate solution (Figure 36-2), which has been associated with lower blood stream infection rates than povidine-iodine or alcohol-based preparations. The skin and tissue around the vessel should be infiltrated with 1% lidocaine solution, except in patients with a known allergy to lidocaine, in whom alternative local anesthetics can be used.
  - Hygiene: The operator should observe proper hand hygiene and use maximal barrier precautions including gown, mask, and gloves and a large sterile drape or multiple drapes covering a large area (Figure 36-3).
- Methods (see Chapter 34 on vessel cannulation).
  - Direct cannulation is typically used for subclavian cannulation.
  - Transfixion may be used for internal jugular and femoral cannulation.
  - Small gauge finder needle to identify vessel location (Figure 36-4).

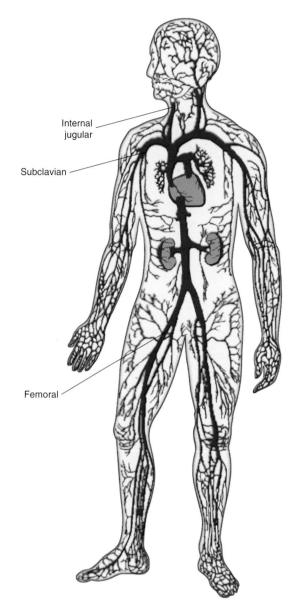

Figure 36-1. Human venous anatomy.

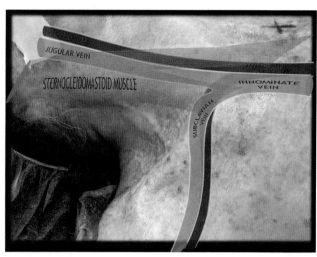

Figure 36-2. Head and neck major vascular anatomy.

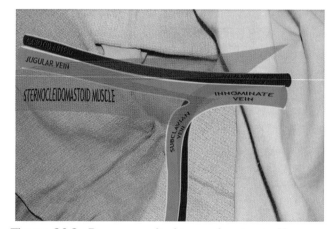

Figure 36-3. Drapes applied to neck prior to IJ cannulation.

Table 36-1. Table showing characteristics of various central venous cannulation sites.

Central Venous Cannulation Sites

Site	Ease of cannulation	Advantages	Disadvantages
Internal jugular	Relatively easy using landmarks and/or ultrasound	Minimal risk of pneumothorax	Risk of carotid artery puncture, infection
Subclavian	Relatively easy using landmarks	Reduced risk of infection	Risk of pneumothorax
Femoral	Easy except in obese patients	Acceptable as a short term vascular access	Risk of infection, decreases patient mobility
Percutaneously inserted central catheter	Difficult, requires specialized skills and equipment (i.e. ultrasound)	Reduced risk of infection	Requires expertise in insertion

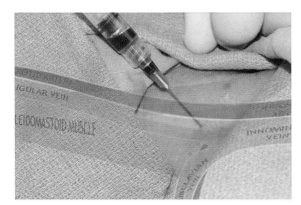

Figure 36-4. Vessel puncture with a "finder" needle.

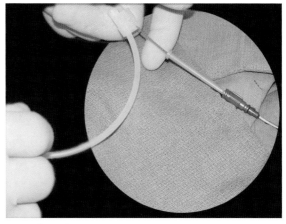

Figure 36-6. Seldinger wire technique—through catheter.

—Seldinger technique can be used as an adjunct for catheter exchange with either of the above cannulation techniques (Figures 36-5 and 36-6).

—Ultrasound-guided vessel location and cannulation has been advocated for internal jugular cannulation and is equally appropriate for femoral cannulation.

▪ The cannulation site should be below the level of the heart during vessel cannulation during IJ and SCV cannulation to prevent air entrainment, and needles and catheter lumens occluded with a finger or obturator.

▪ Many experts recommend transduction of vascular pressure prior to passage of a large bore catheter into the vessel to prevent inadvertent cannulation of a major artery.

▪ Complications.

—Air embolism, which should be treated by positioning patient in left lateral decubitis position, aspiration of air from the vessel, and administration of 100% oxygen to speed reabsorption of the gas

—Pneumothorax

—Arterial puncture

—Delayed complications include infection and thrombosis

▪ A chest x-ray should be obtained following CVC to determine the position of the catheter tip and identify pneumothorax.

 Clinical Pearls and Pitfalls

▪ It may be appropriate to change a preexisting CVC over a wire using a Seldinger technique (Figures 36-7 to 36-10).

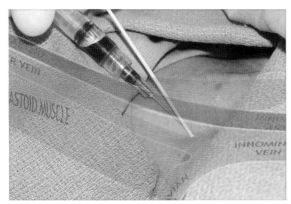

Figure 36-5. Catheter over needle puncture adjacent to finder needle.

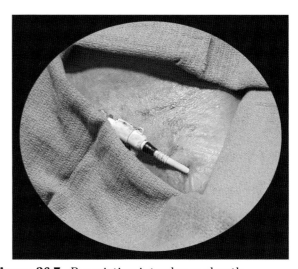

Figure 36-7. Preexisting introducer sheath.

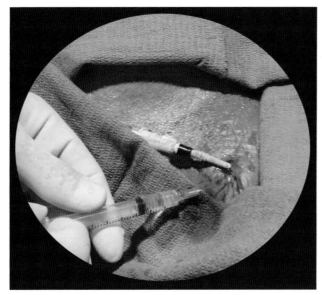

Figure 36-8. Local anesthetic instilled into tissue around introducer sheath.

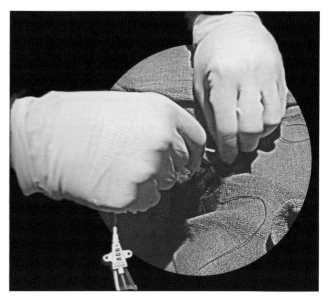

Figure 36-10. New catheter passed over Seldinger wire.

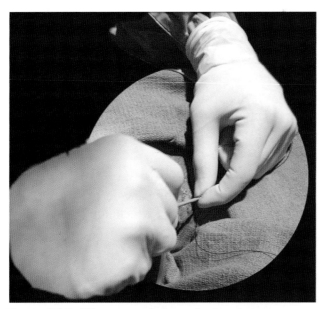

Figure 36-9. Wire passed through sheath for Seldinger catheter exchange.

- In the event of inadvertent arterial puncture, it is appropriate to hold pressure over the site for several minutes and then resume attempts to cannulate the vein.

- Some operators use ultrasound guidance on all cannulation attempts, but ultrasound should be used when repeated anatomically guided attempts have been unsuccessful—ultrasound may identify small, occluded or vessels with an aberrant course.

 Suggested Reading

McGee D.C., Gould M.K. Current concepts: preventing complications of central venous catheterization. *N Engl J Med.* 2003;348(12):1123–1133.

CHAPTER 37

Peripherally Inserted Central Catheter

 Introduction

A peripherally inserted central catheter (PICC) is a relatively new form of central line inserted peripherally, threaded into a central location (Figure 37-1) intended for long-term, including outpatient, use. It is often used for administration of agents such as chemotherapeutic drugs, antibiotics, and parenteral nutrition, and may be associated with a lower rate of infection than centrally inserted catheters.

 Definitions and Terms

- Cephalic vein: travels over the anterior surface of the bicep muscle

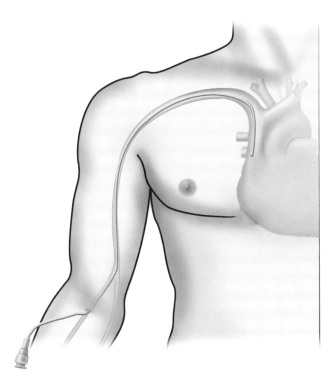

Figure 37-1. Diagrammatic representation of the course of a PICC.

- Basilic vein: travels along the medial aspect of the biceps muscle
- Brachial vein: travels along the medial surface of the forearm
- PICC: PICC line

 Techniques

- Indications for PICC.
  —Intended long-term need for central access
  —Unavailability of other central sites
- Contraindications.
  —Infected over or around intended site
  —Coagulopathy
  —History of axillary node dissection above intended site
  —Radiation above intended site
  —History deep venous thrombosis in veins proximal to intended site
  —Vascular surgery (ie, dialysis access) proximal to intended site
- Prior to procedure, obtain patient consent, prep and drape, and perform universal protocol as described in Section I.
- Identify cannulation site based on patient anatomy and clinical situation.
- Preparation.
  —Skin: The CDC recommends preparation of the cannulation site with a 2% aqueous chlorhexidine-gluconate solution (Figure 37-2), which has been associated with lower blood stream infection rates than povidine-iodine or alcohol-based preparations. The skin and tissue around the vessel should be infiltrated with 1% lidocaine solution, except in patients with a known allergy to lidocaine, in whom alternative local anesthetics can be used.
  —Hygiene: The operator should observe proper hand hygiene and use maximal barrier precautions

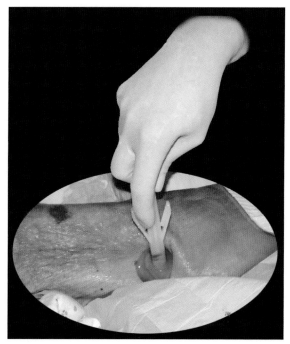

Figure 37-2. Site preparation.

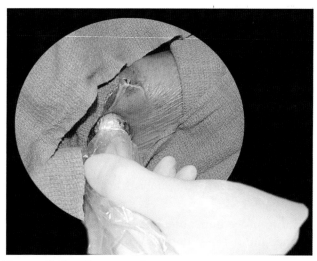

Figure 37-3. Ultrasound probe over antecubital fossa.

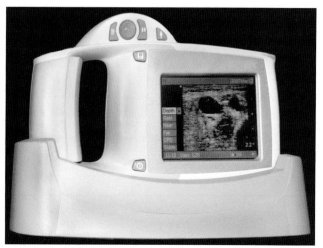

Figure 37-4. Ultrasound image of vessels of interest.

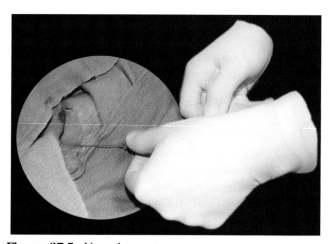

Figure 37-5. Vessel puncture.

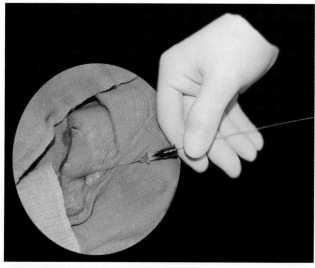

Figure 37-6. Wire through needle.

including gown, mask and gloves, and a large sterile drape or multiple drapes covering a large area.

- Ultrasound (Figures 37-3 and 37-4) is used to identify a patent peripheral vein.
- A small bore needle is inserted into the vessel into which a wire is threaded, followed by a dilator/tear-away sheath combination (Figures 37-5 to 37-8).
- The dilator is removed from the sheath and the PICC catheter is threaded over the wire into the central circulation (Figures 37-9 to 37-11).

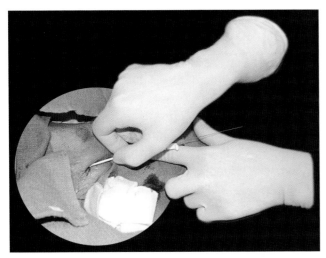

Figure 37-7. Sheath and dilator over wire into vessel.

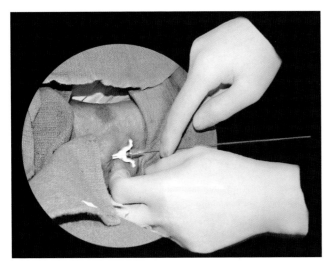

Figure 37-8. Sheath and dilator in vessel.

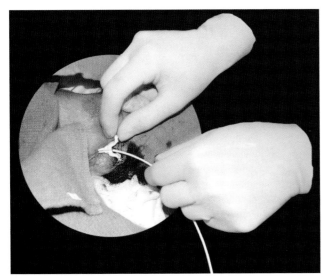

Figure 37-9. Catheter threaded over wire into sheath after removal of dilator.

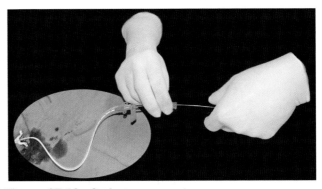

Figure 37-10. Catheter over wire.

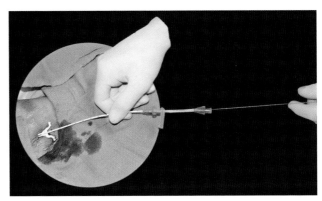

Figure 37-11. Catheter entering thorax.

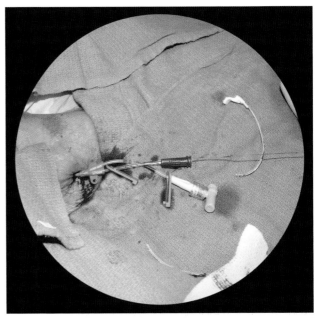

Figure 37-12. Catheter in situ after sheath peeled off.

- The sheath is then peeled away and the wire removed, leaving the PICC in the vessel alone (Figure 37-12).
- A chest x-ray is obtained to confirm the central location of the catheter tip (Figure 37-13).

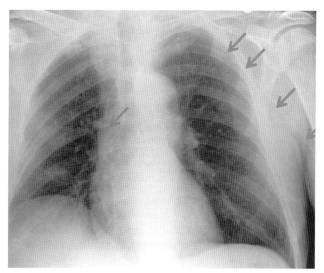

Figure 37-13. Confirmatory x-ray showing the course of catheter and tip in right atrium.

- Complications.
  - —Phlebitis
  - —Catheter occlusion
  - —Catheter fracture

 Clinical Pearls and Pitfalls

- PICC lines can be used to measure CVP although waveforms may be damped due to the length of the catheter.

- PICC lines can be used for bolus administration of drugs, but are not well suited to rapid volume infusion to the combination of their length and small lumen, which increases resistance to rapid fluid flow.

 Suggested Reading

Robinson MK, Mogensen KM, Grudinskas GF, Kohler S, Jacobs DO. Improved care and reduced costs for patients requiring peripherally inserted central catheters: the role of bedside ultrasound and a dedicated team. *J Parenter Enteral Nutr.* 2005;29: 374–379.

CHAPTER 38

Pulmonary Artery Catheterization

Introduction

Pulmonary artery catheterization is a procedure permitting evaluation of pulmonary arterial pressures, pulmonary artery occlusion pressure, cardiac output, mixed venous oxygen saturation, and volumetric measurements on the right side of the heart.

Definitions and Terms

- Pulmonary artery catheter (PAC): A multilumen, balloon-tipped catheter designed to permit simultaneous measurements of pressure in the vena cava and pulmonary artery, as well as intermitted measurement of pulmonary artery occlusion pressure (also called pulmonary capillary wedge pressure) when the balloon is inflated, and measurement of the blood temperature at the tip of the catheter.

- Mixed venous PAC: A PAC equipped with a fiberoptic bundle and designed to permit oximetric analysis of blood at the tip of the catheter—typically in the pulmonary circulation.

- Continuous cardiac output PAC: A PAC equipped with a heating element permitting continuous evaluation of cardiac output.

- Volumetric PAC: A PAC designed to measure right ventricular ejection fraction.

Techniques

- Indications (this is a subject of a great deal of dispute in recent medical literature, so these indications will be very limited in scope):
- —Measurement of pulmonary arterial pressures
- —Direct measurement of cardiac output
- —Continuous measurement of cardiac output and/or mixed venous oxygen saturation

- —Continuous measurement of trends in hemodynamic data
- Contraindications:
- —Coagulopathy
- —Friable right heart lesions (ie, clot or valvular vegetation)
- Access to the central circulation is as described in Chapter 36.
- —The PAC is inserted through an appropriately sized sheath following balloon testing (Figure 38-1) and placement of a sleeve over the PAC (Figure 38-2), which will permit subsequent manipulation of the PAC without surface contamination.
- —The PAC is inserted to a depth of approximately 20 cm, at which point the balloon is inflated (Figure 38-3).
- —The PAC is then advanced through the right ventricle into the pulmonary artery, using waveforms to determine the location of the tip (Figures 38-4 to 38-11).

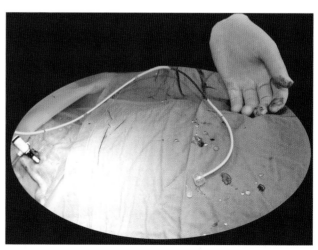

Figure 38-1. PAC prior to insertion laid out with balloon inflated on large drape.

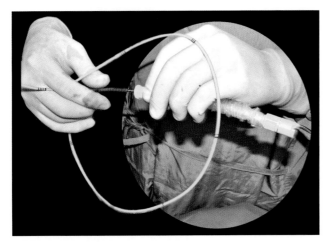

Figure 38-2. Sheath threaded over PAC.

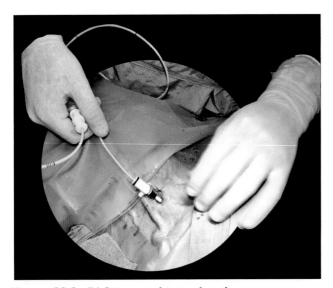

Figure 38-3. PAC inserted into sheath.

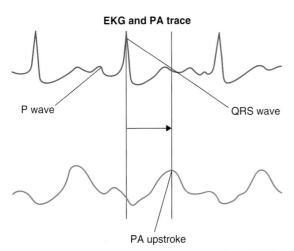

Figure 38-4. Timing of electrocardiographic (ECG) events relative to pulmonary arterial pressure events.

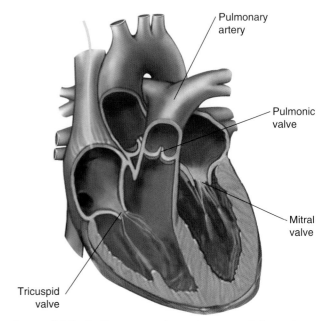

Figure 38-5. Balloon tip advancing into right atrium.

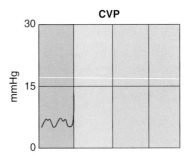

Figure 38-6. Pressure trace corresponding to Figure 38-5.

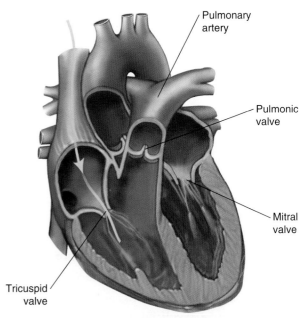

Figure 38-7. Balloon tip advancing into right ventricle.

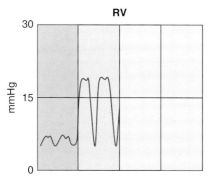

Figure 38-8. Pressure trace corresponding to Figure 38-7.

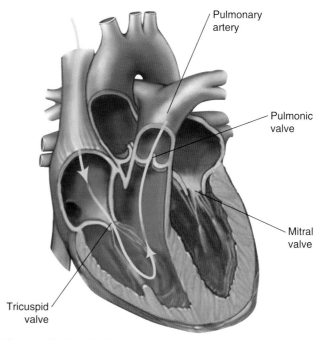

Figure 38-11. Balloon tip in proximal pulmonary artery.

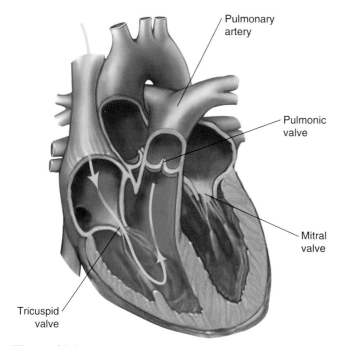

Figure 38-9. Balloon tip approaching pulmonic valve.

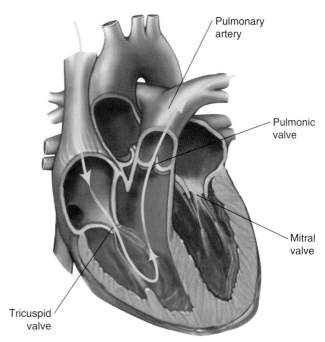

Figure 38-12. Balloon tip in wedge position.

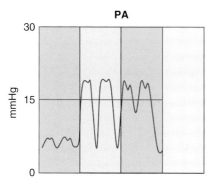

Figure 38-10. Pressure trace corresponding to Figure 38-9.

—When the waveform indicates that balloon is wedged (Figures 38-12 and 38-13), it should be deflated and the sleeve extended to cover the catheter and locked in place.

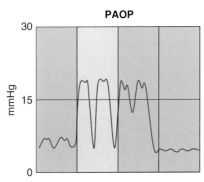

Figure 38-13. Pressure trace corresponding to Figure 38-12.

- Complications:
  —See Chapter 36
  —Pulmonary infarction secondary to prolonged balloon inflation or overinflation
  —Knotting of catheter

 Clinical Pearls and Pitfalls

- The catheter may be difficult to pass for a variety of reasons, including:
  —Tricuspid regurgitation
  —Pulmonic regurgitation
  —Enlarged and/or hypocontractile right ventricle
  —Clot
  —Pacer wires or the presence of other catheters (ie, peripherally inserted central catheters [PICC]) in the vessels or the heart

- Waveforms may be confusing or inaccurate for a variety of reasons, including:
  —Tricuspid or pulmonic regurgitation
  —Intracardiac shunt
  —Air in lines
- PAC passage may precipitate ventricular ectopy or bundle branch block—extreme caution should be used when passing a PAC in a patient with left bundle branch block, who are at risk should the right bundle become injured—it is advisable to have ready access to an external pacer in these patients.

 Suggested Reading

Sandham JD, Hull RD, Brant RF, Knox L, Pineo GF, Doig CJ. A randomized, controlled trial of the use of pulmonary-artery catheters in high-risk surgical patients. *N Engl J Med.* 2003;348(1):5–14.

Richard C, Warszawski J, Anguel N, Deye N, Combes A, Barnoud D. Early use of the pulmonary artery catheter and outcomes in patients with shock and acute respiratory distress syndrome: a randomized controlled trial. *JAMA.* 2003;290(20):2713–2720.

Rhodes A, Cusack RJ, Newman PJ. A randomised, controlled trial of the pulmonary artery catheter in critically ill patients. *Intensive Care Med.* 2002;28(3): 256–264.

Harvey S, Harrison DA, Singer M, Ashcroft J, Jones CM, Elbourne D. Assessment of the clinical effectiveness of pulmonary artery catheters in management of patients in intensive care (PAC-Man): a randomised controlled trial. *Lancet.* 2005;366(9484):472–477.

CHAPTER 39

Cardiac Output Determination

Introduction

Cardiac output (CO) can be determined by indicator dilution (typically thermodilution), where CO is a function of the quantity of the indicator divided by the area under the dilution curve as measured at a downstream location. In practice, a bolus of cold fluid is injected into the circulation in the vena cava through the pulmonary artery catheter (PAC) and the area is measured under the temperature-change curve in the pulmonary circulation at the PAC balloon tip. This chapter will describe the bolus method to characterize the general technique of thermodilution, although continuous CO measurement is increasingly prevalent.

Definitions and Terms

- Thermodilution: Measurement of blood flow in the circulation based on an induced change in the heat content of blood flowing downstream from the heat change.

- Thermistor: A temperature sensing resistor integrated into a PAC.

- Bolus CO: In which a bolus of indicator (typically cold saline) is injected into the circulation as the indicator.

- Continuous CO: In which the blood is heat in pulses upstream of the thermistor and CO is determined by a mathematical transformation using the heat current changes (continuous cardiac output calculation is performed automatically by a computer attached to the pulmonary arterial catheter).

- Fick method: An approach to calculating CO relying on assumptions about patient systemic oxygen consumption, using the following formula:

  —Cardiac out put = ((125 mL/min oxygen × body surface area (m²)/(arteriovenous oxygen difference)) × 100

Techniques

- Manual thermodilution bolus CO:

  —A predetermined bolus (5-10 cc) of saline of known temperature (as based on the measurement of the injectate temperature) is injected into the central venous pressure (CVP) port of PAC (Figures 39-1 and 39-2).

  —A CO-analysis computer characterizes the heat change of the blood at the PAC tip as a curve (Figure 39-3), and the area under the curve is used to calculate CO by dividing that area into the amount of indicator, consequently:

    • Lesser area under the curve is consistent with faster blood flow and higher CO (Figure 39-4).
    • Greater area under the curve is consistent with slower blood flow and lower CO (Figure 39-5).

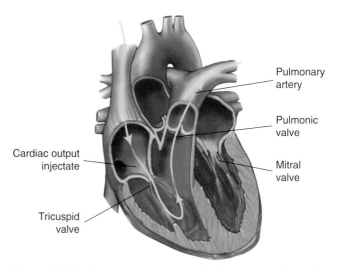

Figure 39-1. Showing injection of indicator in the right atrium or vena cava and flow through the heart.

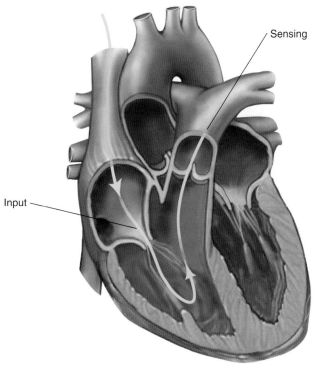

Figure 39-2. Showing injection and sensing of the indicator.

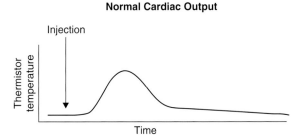

Normal Cardiac Output

Figure 39-3. Shows a normal CO curve (note that although dye temperature may be lower than that of blood, the output curve is typically represented as a temperature curve above the baseline).

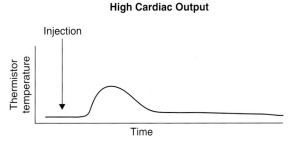

High Cardiac Output

Figure 39-4. Shows a high CO, with correspondingly reduced area under the curve.

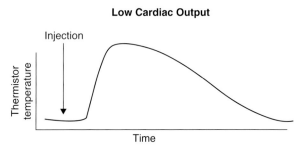

Low Cardiac Output

Figure 39-5. Shows a low CO, with correspondingly increased area under the curve.

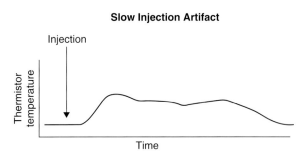

Slow Injection Artifact

Figure 39-6. Shows injection artifact with blunted curve.

—A series of determinations are typically averaged together to determine CO after discarding unreliable measurements (Figure 39-6).

 Clinical Pearls and Pitfalls

- There are a variety of confounders that can invalidate CO analysis, including:
  —Slow or irregular bolus injection
  —Incorrect injectate temperature (ie, the number used in the CO formula for injectate temperature is inaccurate, leading the computer to "think" that the injectate is warmer or colder than it actually is)
  —Tricuspid or pulmonic regurgitation, or intracardiac shunt
- There is a sufficient amount of noise in any CO measurement approach that clinical analysis should typically be based on trended performance rather than absolute value of the CO at any one point in time.

Suggested Reading

Ganz W, Donoso R, Marcus HS, Forrester JS, Swan HJC. A new technique for measurement of cardiac output by thermodilution in man. *Am J Cardiol.* 1971;27:392–396.

Hillis LD, Firth BG, Winniford MD. Analysis of factors affecting the variability of Fick versus indicator dilution measurements of cardiac output. *Am J Cardiol.* 1985;56:764–768.

Kadota LT. Theory and application of thermodilution cardiac output measurement: a review. *Heart Lung.* 1985;14:605–614.

Goldenheim, PD, Kazemi H. Cardiopulmonary monitoring of critically ill patients. *N Engl J Med.* 1984;311: 776–780.

CHAPTER 40

Intra-Aortic Balloon Pump Insertion

Introduction

An intra-aortic balloon pump (IABP) is an electrocardiogram (ECG) synchronized endovascular balloon that inflates in the proximal descending aorta (Figure 40-1) during cardiac diastole, acting both to augment coronary perfusion and cardiac output, and deflates during systole, permitting cardiac ejection.

Definitions and Terms

- Counterpulsation: Rhythmic mechanical pumping synchronized with the heartbeat.
- Systole: The phase of the heartbeat during which cardiac muscle contracts actively ejecting blood through the open aortic valve.

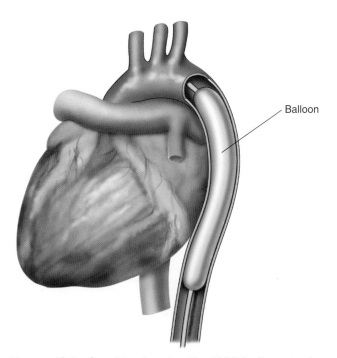

Figure 40-1. Graphic showing the IABP balloon in the proximal descending aorta.

- Diastole: The phase of the heartbeat during which the left ventricle fills with blood from the left atrium through the open mitral valve, and during which the majority of coronary perfusion occurs.

Techniques

- Indications:
  - Unstable angina
  - Cardiogenic shock
  - Cardiac insufficiency following cardiac surgery
  - Mechanical cardiac support in the setting of certain cardiac lesions such as acute mitral insufficiency or intracardiac shunt
- Contraindications:
  - Aortic dissection
  - Aortic insufficiency
  - Severe atherosclerotic disease of the aorta
  - Aortic aneurysm
  - Aortic graft
- Prior to procedure, obtain patient consent, prep and drape, and perform universal protocol as described in Section I.
- The IABP is almost invariably placed through one of the femoral arteries.
- Preparation:
  - Skin: The Center for Disease Control and Prevention (CDC) recommends preparation of the cannulation site with a 2% aqueous chlorhexidine-gluconate solution, which has been associated with lower blood stream infection rates than povidone-iodine or alcohol-based preparations. The skin and tissue around the vessel should be infiltrated with 1% lidocaine solution, except in patients with a known allergy to lidocaine, in whom alternative local anesthetics can be used.

—Hygiene: The operator should observe proper hand-hygiene and use maximal barrier precautions including gown, mask and gloves, and a large sterile drape or multiple drapes covering a large area.

- Methods (see Chapter 34 on vessel cannulation):

—Direct cannulation.

—Transfixion.

—Seldinger technique is used as an adjunct for catheter exchange with either of the above cannulation techniques.

—Ultrasound guided vessel location can be used for femoral cannulation.

- Following access to the vessel, the IABP is inserted to a premeasured depth so as to lie in the proximal descending aorta (Figures 40-2 to 40-5).

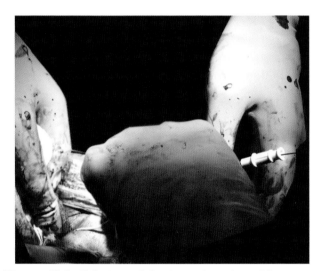

Figure 40-2. Dilation of the insertion site with a dilator over a wire in the vessel.

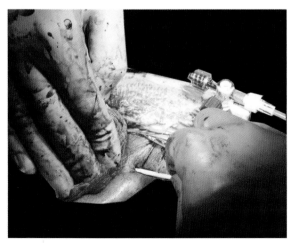

Figure 40-3. Dilation with a larger sheath.

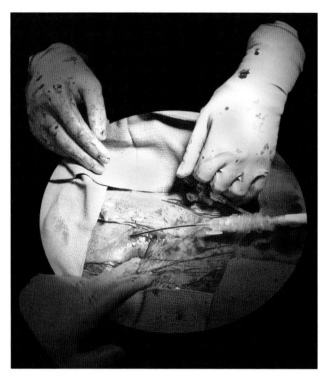

Figure 40-4. Balloon inserted into the vessel.

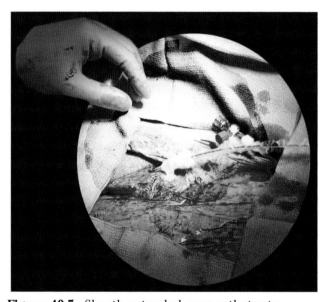

Figure 40-5. Sheath extended over catheter to permit sterile balloon repositioning.

- Balloon inflation is timed to occur during diastole, and gated to the ECG or arterial pulse wave (Figure 40-6).
- The pumping ratio is typically 1:1, although it may be reduced to 1:2 and/or 1:3 prior to removal.

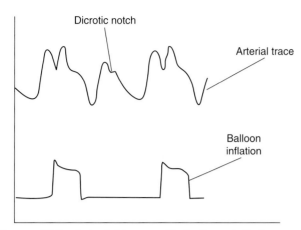

Figure 40-6. Arterial trace with balloon inflation timed during diastole at a 1:2 ratio.

- A confirmatory chest x-ray is used to identify the location of the tip of the balloon.
- Complications are varied, and include:
  —Leg ischemia or compartment syndrome
  —Aortic dissection
  —Embolization of debris to the brain and/or visceral organs

 Clinical Pearls and Pitfalls

- Triggering may be difficult with irregular heart rhythms or at a high rate, and a 1:2 triggering ratio may be appropriate if tolerated by patient (Figure 40-7).
- Pulses and perfusion distal to the IABP insertion site should be closely monitored for signs of ischemia.

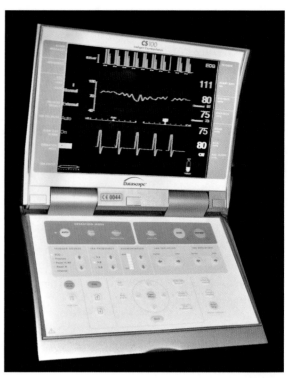

Figure 40-7. IABP console with ECG and balloon inflation timed at a 1:2 ratio.

 Suggested Reading

Boehmer JP, Popjes E. Cardiac failure: mechanical support strategies. *Crit Care Med.* 2006;34(suppl 9): S268–S277.

Bates ER, Stomel RJ, Hochman JS, Ohman EM. The use of intraaortic balloon counterpulsation as an adjunct to reperfusion therapy in cardiogenic shock. *Int J Cardiol.* 1998;65(suppl 1):S37–S42.

CHAPTER 41

Pericardiocentesis

 Introduction

Pericardiocentesis is performed to remove fluid from the pericardium for diagnostic purposes or as a therapy for pericardial tamponade.

 Definitions and Terms

- Pericardial tamponade: Clinical scenario in which fluid accumulates in the pericardial sac to the point that pericardial pressure impedes venous return to the heart—this may occur acutely as with an injury to the heart or chronically, wherein a large amount of fluid accumulates over time.
- Pericardial effusion: Accumulation of fluid in the pericardial sac.

 Techniques

- Indications for pericardiocentesis:
  - Pericardial tamponade
  - Pericardial effusion
  - Pericardial fluid drainage where purulent effusion suspected
  - Diagnosis of etiology for effusion
- Contraindications:
  - Coagulopathy.
  - Small or loculated effusion, where surgery is the preferred alternative.
  - Prior to procedure, obtain patient consent, prep and drape, and perform universal protocol as described in Section I.
  - Identify drainage site based on echocardiography or fluoroscopy.
- Preparation:
  - Skin: The Center for Disease Control and Prevention (CDC) recommends preparation of the cannulation site with a 2% aqueous chlorhexidine-gluconate solution, which has been associated with lower blood stream infection rates than povidone-iodine or alcohol-based preparations. The skin and tissue around over the site should be infiltrated with 1% lidocaine solution, except in patients with a known allergy to lidocaine, in whom alternative local anesthetics can be used.
  - Hygiene: The operator should observe proper hand hygiene and use maximal barrier precautions including gown, mask and gloves, and a large sterile drape or multiple drapes covering a large area.
- Methods:
  - Position patient with head of bed elevated to pool effusion in the dependent portion of the pericardial sac.
  - A sterile electrocardiograph (ECG) lead should be attached to the pericardiocentesis needle (which may be a spinal needle).
  - The needle is inserted under the xiphoid at a 20° angle to the skin and directed toward the left shoulder (Figure 41-1).
  - The ECG is monitored continuously for injury current as the needle is advanced.
  - The needle is advanced until there is fluid return or an injury current (ST elevation) on the ECG.
  - If fluid is aspirated, a flexible guidewire is inserted through the needle into the effusion.

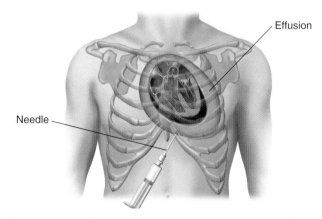

Figure 41-1. Graphic showing anatomic approach to pericardiocentesis.

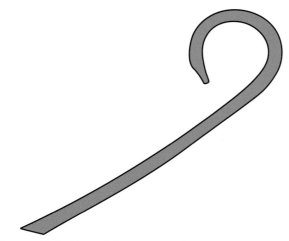

Figure 41-2. Pigtail drainage catheter.

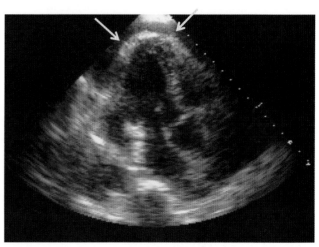

Figure 41-3. Transthoracic echocardiogram showing pericardial effusion beneath transducer head.

—The needle is then withdrawn and a pigtail catheter (Figure 41-2) inserted over the wire and secured in place if the catheter is to be left in place.

—Fluid is then drained from the pericardium and sent for diagnostic studies as indicated.

▪Complications:

—Pericardial tamponade

—Coronary artery or vein laceration

—Cardiac ectopy

—Pneumothorax

 ## Clinical Pearls and Pitfalls

▪So-called "blind" pericardiocentesis can be performed in the event of an emergency, but echocardiographically guided procedures are preferable (Figure 41-3).

▪Echo contrast (saline agitated with air) can be injected into pericardial space during echocardiographic visualization to confirm correct needle or catheter position in the pericardial space.

 ## Suggested Reading

Tsang TS, Enriquez-Sarano M, Freeman WK, Barnes ME, Sinak LJ, Gersh BJ. Consecutive 1127 therapeutic echocardiographically guided pericardiocenteses: clinical profile, practice patterns, and outcomes spanning 21 years. *Mayo Clin Proc.* 2002;77:429–436.

Bastian A, Meissner A, Lins M, et al. Pericardiocentesis: differential aspects of a common procedure. *Intensive Care Med.* 2000;26:572–576.

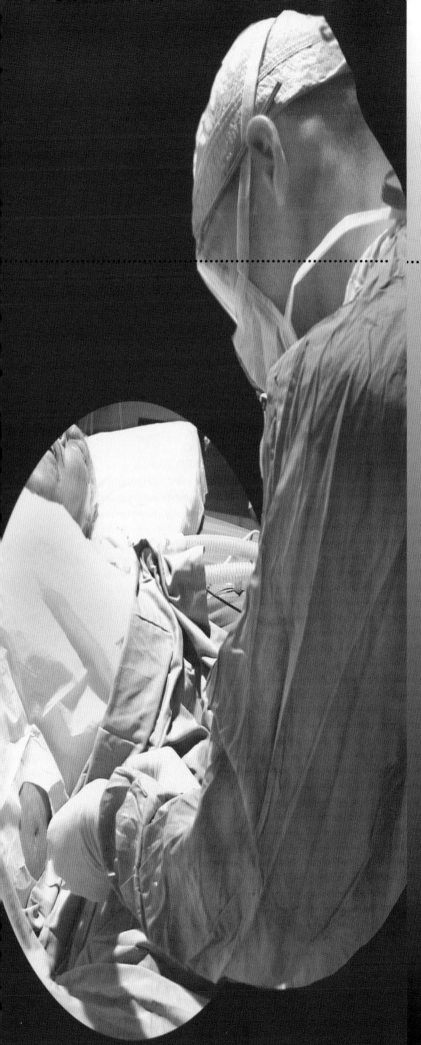

SECTION V

Gastrointestinal Features

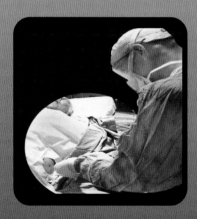

CHAPTER 42

Nasogastric Tube Insertion

Introduction

A nasogastric tube is inserted in the intensive care unit (ICU) for a variety of reasons including gastric emptying, drainage, and feeding.

Definitions and Terms

- Nasogastric tube (NG): A tube passing through the nose, pharynx, and esophagus, with the distal tip in the stomach.

Techniques

- Indications:
  —Nasogastric drainage in various setting:
    • Ileus
    • Following abdominal surgery
    • To prevent regurgitation
  —Administration of certain drugs directly into the stomach:
    • Activated charcoal in the event of a drug ingestion
  —Diagnosis of ingested substance (ie, when it is unclear what patient has ingested).
  —Enteral feeding:
    • In a patient with an endotracheal tube.
    • In a patient who is unable to protect airway.
- Contraindications:
  —Coagulopathy
  —Sinusitis
  —Head trauma
  —Esophageal surgery or stricture
  —Deviated septum
- Technique:
  —When possible identify more patent nasal passage by having patient sniff through each nasal passage.
  —Position patient:

• If awake, the patient should be placed in a head-up position.

• If unconscious, the patient should be placed in a supine position.

—Lubricate NG tube and advance into nose, aiming for the ear.

—As tip of tube passes into nasopharynx, encourage awake patient to swallow to facilitate passage of tube into esophagus—it may be appropriate to have patient drink through straw during the procedure.

—Advance tube to premeasured depth corresponding to mid gastric position of the tip (Figure 42-1).

—Verify tube position by aspiration of gastric contents, audible bubbling on auscultation over stomach when air injected into tube, and/or abdominal flat plate x-ray (Figure 42-2).

—Secure NG tube to nose with tape.

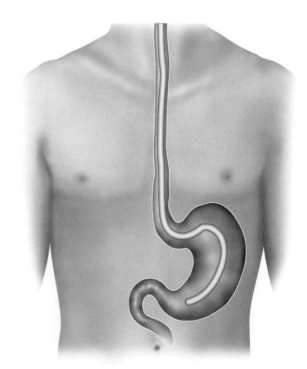

Figure 42-1. Graphic showing NG tube position in stomach.

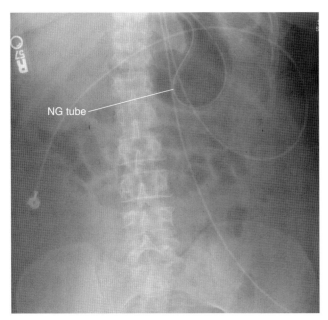

Figure 42-2. Abdominal flat plat showing NG tube coiled in stomach.

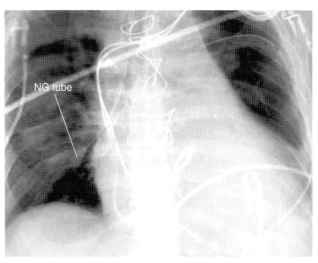

Figure 42-3. Chest x-ray showing NG tube in right lung.

- Complications
  - —Epistaxis:
  - —Perforation of cribriform plate
  - —Esophageal perforation
  - —Tracheal intubation with NG tube (Figure 42-3)
  - —Pneumothorax

 ## Clinical Pearls and Pitfalls

- NG tube should be very well lubricated to prevent mucosal abrasion.

- Patient should be able to speak following placement—if unable, NG tube may be between vocal cords.

- In unconscious patients, tube insertion may be guided with fingers, laryngoscopy, or laryngeal manipulation.

- Do not tape tube too tightly to nose to prevent alar injury.

 ## Suggested Reading

Thomsen TW, Shaffer RW, Setnik G. Videos in clinical medicine. Nasogastric intubation. *N Engl J Med.* 2006;354:e16.

CHAPTER 43

Nasoduodenal Feeding Tube

 ## Introduction

Enteral feeding may be performed using a standard nasogastric or a nasoduodenal tube. The latter is a small bore tube advanced through the stomach, into the duodenum, and used specifically for feeding.

 ## Definitions and Terms

- Postpyloric tube: Nasal feeding tube with the distal type beyond the pyloric valve—typically in the duodenum.
- Nasoenteric tube: Tube passing through the nose into the gut.

 ## Techniques

- Indications:
  —Long-term enteral feeding in a patient who requires total or supplementary enteral feeding, and for whom gastric feeding is inappropriate.
- Contraindications:
  —Coagulopathy
  —Sinusitis
  —Head trauma
  —Esophageal surgery or stricture
  —Deviated septum
- Technique:
  —When possible identify more patent nasal passage by having patient sniff through each nasal passage.
  —Position patient:
  - If awake, the patient should be placed in a head-up position.
  - If unconscious, the patient should be placed in a supine position.
  —Nasoduodenal tubes are typically narrow, flexible (Figure 43-1), and equipped with a wire to stiffen

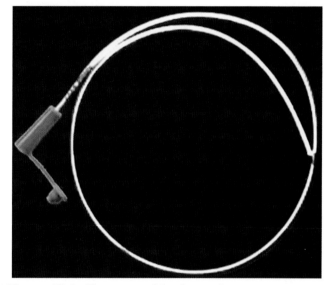

Figure 43-1. Nasoenteral feeding tube.

tube during passage, which is subsequently removed—the tip may be weighted to facilitate tube advancement.

—Fluoroscopic assistance may be used to facilitate correct positioning of tube (Figure 43-2).

—Lubricate enteral tube and advance into nose, aiming for the ear (Figures 43-3 and 43-4).

—As the tip of the tube passes into nasopharynx, encourage awake patient to swallow to facilitate passage of tube into esophagus—it may be appropriate to have patient drink through a straw during the procedure.

—Advance tube to premeasured depth corresponding to gastric position of tip.

—Verify tube position by audible bubbling on auscultation over stomach when air injected into tube and/or abdominal flat plate x-ray (Figure 43-5).

—Secure nasogastric tube (NG) tube to nose with tape.

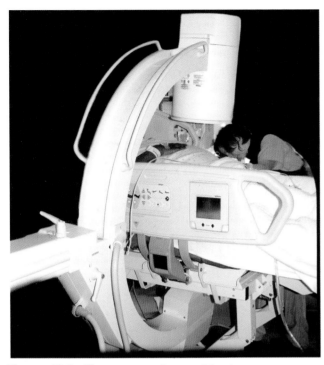

Figure 43-2. Fluoroscope for positioning.

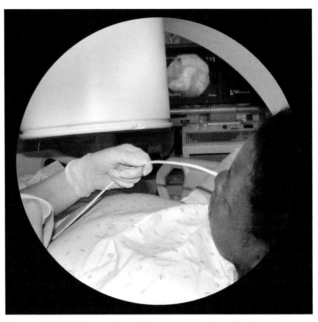

Figure 43-4. Insertion of nasoenteric tube into nose.

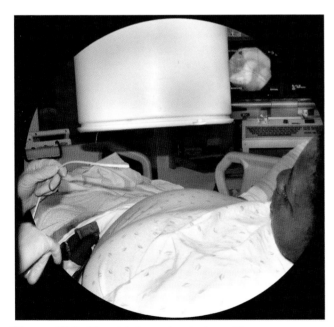

Figure 43-3. Nasal tube prior to insertion.

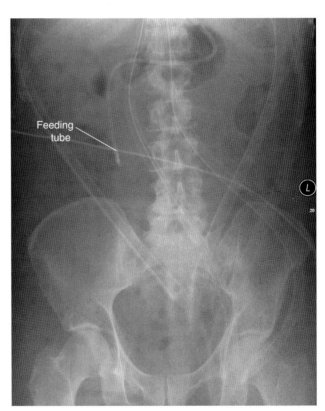

Feeding
tube

Figure 43-5. Abdominal x-ray showing post-pyloric position of feeding tube tip.

▪ Complications:

—Epistaxis

—Perforation of cribriform plate

—Esophageal perforation

—Tracheal intubation with NG tube (Figure 43-6)

—Pneumothorax

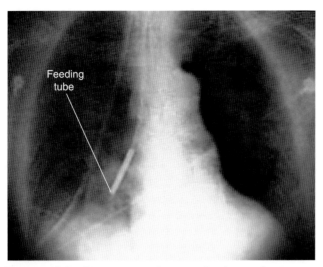

Figure 43-6. Chest x-ray showing feeding tube in right lower lobe.

Clinical Pearls and Pitfalls

- When the tube is positioned in stomach but the tip cannot be advanced manually past pyloric valve, a promotility agent such as erythromycin may be administered to encourage gastric propulsion of tube tip into duodenum.
- Nasoduodenal feeds are typically administered continuously as contrasted with bolus NG tube feeds, where residual volumes are check periodically.

Suggested Reading

Ho KM, Dobb GJ, Webb SA. A comparison of early gastric and post-pyloric feeding in critically ill patients: a meta-analysis. *Intensive Care Med.* 2006;32:639–649.

de Aguilar-Nascimento JE, Kudsk KA. Use of small-bore feeding tubes: successes and failures. *Curr Opin Clin Nutr Metab Care.* 2007;10:291–296.

CHAPTER 44

Percutaneous Gastric Tube

 ## Introduction

Percutaneously placed endogastric tubes can be placed in suitable patients in the intensive care unit (ICU) with the guidance of a gastroscope.

 ## Definitions and Terms

- Percutaneous endoscopic gastrostomy (PEG): PEG tube (Figure 44-1).
- Pull technique: An approach whereby the feeding tube is pulled from the stomach out through the abdominal wall under endoscopic guidance.
- Push technique: An approach whereby the feeding tube is pulled through the abdominal wall from the skin surface into the stomach, again under endoscopic guidance.

 ## Techniques

- Indications:
  - Requirement for long-term enteral feeding in a patient who is unable to sustain adequate caloric intake by mouth.

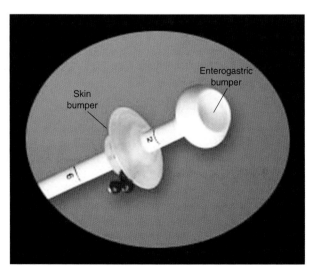

Figure 44-1. PEG tube.

- Contraindications:
  - Coagulopathy
  - Unfavorable gastric anatomy
  - Gastric pathology
    - Neoplasm
    - Varices
    - Gastritis
  - Abdominal wall infection or burn
  - Previous gastric or intra-abdominal surgery
- Technique:
  - This procedure requires the participation of a skilled endoscopist.
  - Prior to the procedure, patient consent should be obtained, skin should be prepped and draped, and universal protocol should be performed as per Section I.
  - A gastroscope is introduced into the stomach, entire content of the stomach is suctioned out, air insufflated to distend abdomen and the endoscopic light is used to transilluminate the anterior abdominal wall.
  - The skin is anesthetized over the point of maximal light.
  - An Angiocath is pushed through skin into stomach.
    - Pull technique:
      - Guidewire is introduced through the Angiocath and pulled out through the mouth, where it is attached to feeding tube.
      - The PEG tube is then pulled back into stomach and out through abdominal wall and secured (Figure 44-2).
    - Push technique:
      - Guidewire introduced into stomach through Angiocath and a series of dilators are used with Seldinger technique to dilate gastrostomy.
      - The PEG tube is then pushed into stomach over wire and secured.
- Complications:
  - Cellulitis

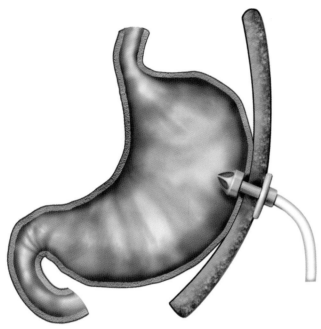

Figure 44-2. Graphic showing PEG tube in position.

—Pneumoperitoneum

—Gastroenteric fistula

—Bowel peroration with peritonitis

—Device malposition

 ## Clinical Pearls and Pitfalls

▪ Gastroscopically guided procedure should be abandoned if the anterior stomach wall does not transilluminate—this indicates that there is some organ or other impediment (ie, ascites, scars) to passage of needle directly through skin into stomach wall.

 ## Suggested Reading

Gopalan S, Khanna S. Enteral nutrition delivery technique. *Curr Opin Clin Nutr Metab Care.* 2003;6:313–317.

Pennington C. To PEG or not to PEG. *Clin Med.* 2002;2:250–255.

Pearce CB, Duncan HD. Enteral feeding. Nasogastric, nasojejunal, percutaneous endoscopic gastrostomy, or jejunostomy: its indications and limitations. *Postgrad Med J.* 2002;78:198–204.

CHAPTER 45

Paracentesis

 Introduction

Paracentesis is performed in the intensive care unit (ICU) for diagnostic or therapeutic purposes to drain free fluid from the peritoneum.

 Definitions and Terms

- Paracentesis: Aspiration of peritoneal fluid from the abdomen (Figure 45-1).
- Peritoneal lavage: To be distinguished from paracentesis—performed to evaluate abdomen for free bleeding typically following trauma—has been largely supplemented by ultrasound.

 Techniques

- Indications:
  —Diagnostic:
  - To determine the etiology of ascites.
  - To diagnose infection in chronic ascites (ie, spontaneous bacterial peritonitis).
  - To diagnose intra-abdominal malignancy.
  —Therapeutic:
  - To relieve respiratory distress due to ascites.
  - To decrease intra-abdominal pressure and improve venous return.
- Contraindications:
  —Coagulopathy
  —Acute abdominal process requiring surgical management
  —Skin cellulitis over proposed incision site
  —Distended bladder or bowel
  —Previous abdominal surgery with adhesions
  —Pregnancy
- Ultrasound and/or physical examination (ie, presence of a fluid wave) can be used to diagnose presence and/or location of ascetic fluid.
- Prior to the procedure, patient consent should be obtained, site should be prepped and draped, and universal protocol should be performed as per Section I.
- The bladder and stomach should be emptied prior to performance of the procedure.
- Technique:
  —Patient should be positioned supine or in lateral decubitus position in order to bring free ascites below proposed insertion spot as determined by examination or ultrasound.
  —Local anesthetic is infiltrated into skin over proposed paracentesis site, typically paramedian (Figure 45-2) in anterior axillary line or in midline below umbilicus.
  —A needle or Angiocath is inserted into the abdomen and aspirated (Figures 45-3 and 45-4).
  —When free ascites fluid is obtained, a wire may be introduced into needle or Angiocath according to Seldinger technique, and a catheter introduced over the wire for fluid drainage (Figures 45-5 to 45-9).
  —Samples of the fluid are sent for diagnostic studies as warranted.
- Complications:
  —Gastric or bowel perforation
  —Peritonitis

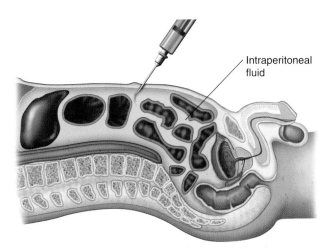

Intraperitoneal fluid

Figure 45-1. Graphic showing paracentesis aspiration of peritoneal fluid.

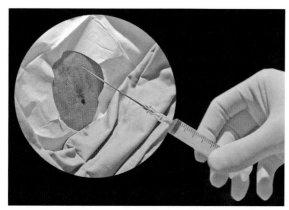

Figure 45-2. Infiltration of local anesthetic in skin wall along anterior axillary line.

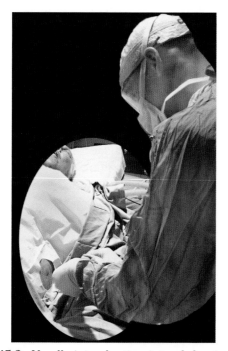

Figure 45-3. Needle introduction into abdominal wall.

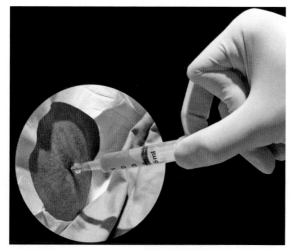

Figure 45-4. Ascitic fluid aspiration.

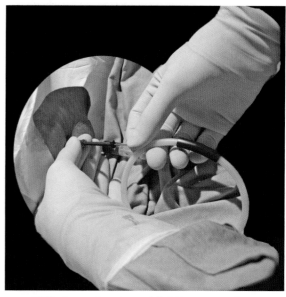

Figure 45-5. Introduction of Seldinger exchange wire through needle into abdomen.

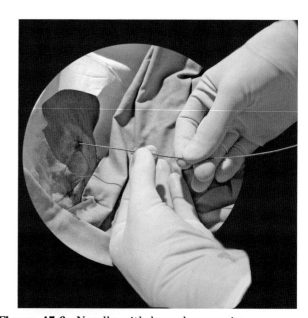

Figure 45-6. Needle withdrawal over wire.

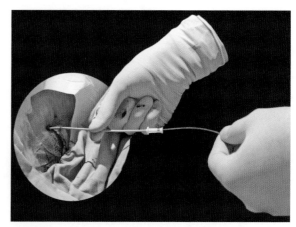

Figure 45-7. Catheter introduction over wire.

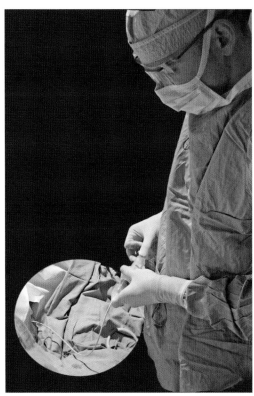

Figure 45-8. Aspiration of ascites fluid through catheter.

—Post-paracentesis hypotension secondary to volume redistribution

—Intra-abdominal bleeding

 Clinical Pearls and Pitfalls

▪In patients with tense ascites, fluid may leak from site following the procedure unless a "z" track is used for needle insertion—alternatively a pursestring suture may be applied around site.

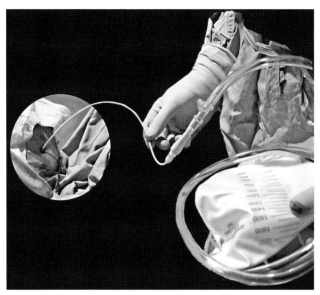

Figure 45-9. Passive drainage of ascites fluid into drainage bag.

▪The patient may be repositioned during fluid drainage to facilitate maximal fluid drainage.

▪Patients with severe liver failure may benefit from colloid administration during or after the procedure to prevent hypotension due to fluid shifts.

▪Patients with cirrhosis may have abdominal varices, and the paracentesis site should avoid visible vessels.

 Suggested Reading

Thomsen TW, Shaffer RW, White B, Setnik GS. Paracentesis. *N Engl J Med.* 2006;355:e21.
Sandhu BS, Sanyal AJ. Management of ascites in cirrhosis. *Clin Liver Dis.* 2005;9:715–732.

CHAPTER 46

Abdominal Compartment Syndrome Diagnosis

Introduction

Abdominal compartment syndrome (ACS) occurs when intra-abdominal pressure increases to the point that it exceeds pressure in the inferior vena cava and prevents venous return to the heart.

Definitions and Terms

- Primary ACS: Accumulation of fluid in the abdomen due to acute intra-abdominal process (Figure 46-1):
  —Penetrating or blunt trauma to the abdomen or pelvis with hemorrhage
  —Abdominal crush injury
  —Intra-abdominal vascular rupture or injury
  —Bowel perforation
  —Pancreatitis
- Secondary ACS: Accumulation of fluid in abdomen without obvious abdominal injury:
  —Large volume fluid resuscitation
  —Postoperative third-spacing of fluid into peritoneum and bowel edema
  —Abdominal packing
  —Sepsis
  —Large area full-thickness burns
- Chronic ACS:
  —Cirrhosis
  —Peritoneal dialysis
  —Meig syndrome

Techniques

- The diagnosis of ACS requires a high index of clinical suspicion in the appropriate clinical setting.
- Diagnosis is typically made by measuring intra-abdominal pressure by transducing bladder pressure.
- Measurement of intra-abdominal pressure:
  —Urinary drainage catheter is clamped.
  —A needle connecting a fluid column to a transducer is introduced through the wall of the catheter and pressure is transduced (Figure 46-2):

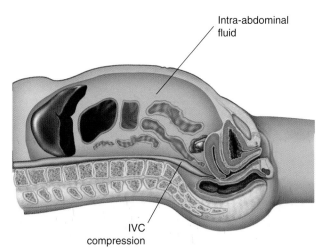

Figure 46-1. Graphic of ACS showing veno-caval compression.

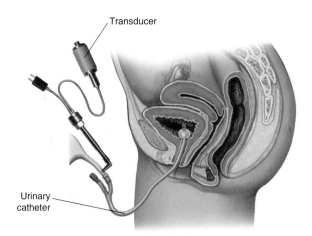

Figure 46-2. Graphic showing bladder pressure measurement as a surrogate for intra-abdominal pressure.

- Grade I ACS: pressure 10 to 15 cm H_2O
- Grade II ACS: pressure 16 to 25 H_2O
- Grade III ACS: pressure 26 to 35 cm H_2O
- Grade IV ACS: pressure > 35 cm H_2O

 ## Clinical Pearls and Pitfalls

- Patients with ACS may have increased airway pressures.
- The diagnoses of pericardial tamponade and tension pneumothorax may be suspected when the patient actually has ACS.

 ## Suggested Reading

Burch JM, Moore EE, Moore FA, Franciose R. The abdominal compartment syndrome. *Surg Clin North Am.* 1996;76:833–842.

Kirkpatrick AW, Balogh Z, Ball CG, et al. The secondary abdominal compartment syndrome: iatrogenic or unavoidable? *J Am Coll Surg.* 2006;202:668–679.

Sugrue M. Abdominal compartment syndrome. *Curr Opin Crit Care.* 2005;11:333–338.

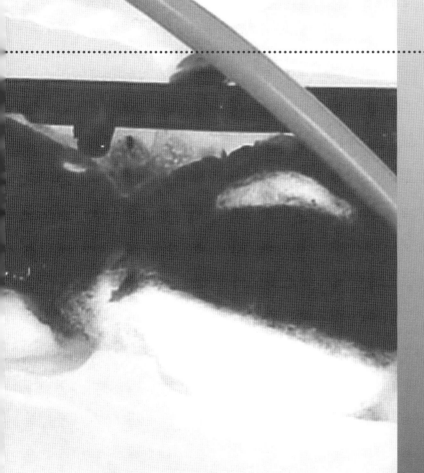

Genitourinary Procedures

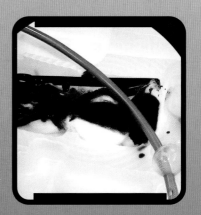

CHAPTER 47

Male Urinary Drainage Catheter

 Introduction

Urinary catheter insertion is performed to drain urine from the bladder (Figure 47-1) in patients who are incontinent or have urinary obstruction or to frequently monitor urine output as a proxy for renal function. Long-term catheterization is associated with increased risk of urinary tract infection.

 Definitions and Terms

- French (Fr): The unit of measurement used in sizing urinary catheters—where 1 French equals 1/3 of a millimeter.
- Intermittent straight catheterization: A technique used for intermittent bladder drainage wherein the catheter is inserted and removed periodically to decompress bladder.
- Prostatic hypertrophy: A common cause of difficulty with spontaneous urinary drainage as well as catheter insertion.

 Techniques

- Indications:
  - Perioperative urinary drainage
  - Urinary tract outflow obstruction
  - Urinary volume measurement in the intensive care unit (ICU)
- Contraindications:
  - Urethral disruption

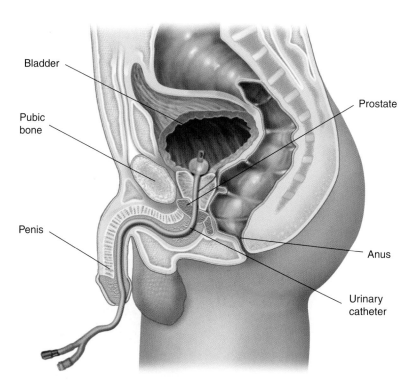

Figure 47-1. Male urinary anatomy.

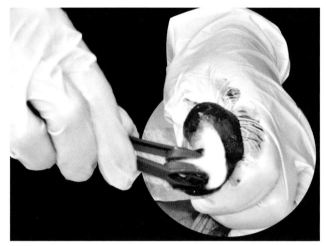

Figure 47-2. Urinary drainage catheter and tested balloon.

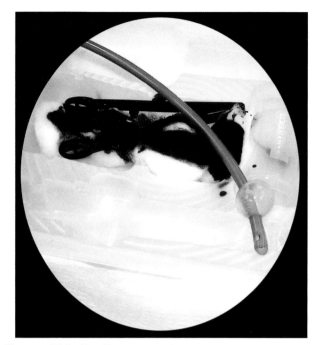

Figure 47-3. Penile preparation.

- Method:
  - —Prior to urinary catheterization, patient consent should be obtained, the urethra and surrounding areas prepped and draped (Figure 47-2), and the universal protocol performed as described in Section I.
  - —Prior to catheterization, the operator should wash hands and wear sterile gloves.
  - —According to Centers for Disease Control guidelines, Catheters should only be inserted by trained personnel.
    - Catheters should only be inserted when necessary, rather than for the convenience of patient-care personnel, and should only be left in place as long as necessary.
    - Alternative methods of urinary drainage should be entertained (ie, condom catheter, suprapubic drain).
  - —The smallest appropriate catheter should be selected for insertion, and the balloon checked for patency (Figure 47-3):
    - Smaller catheters (12-14 Fr) are appropriate for use in patients with strictures.
    - Medium catheters (16-18 Fr) are typically used in adult males.
    - Larger catheters (20-24 Fr) may be used in patients with prostatic hypertrophy or hematuria.
  - —If the patient is uncircumcised, the foreskin should be retracted prior to skin preparation.
  - —The catheter should be lubricated and inserted into the urethra and advance to its full length, while the penis is held vertically with the nondominant hand (Figures 47-4 and 47-5).

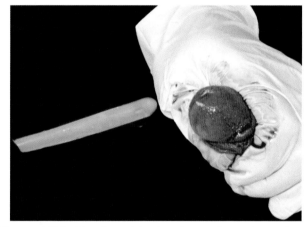

Figure 47-4. Hand positioning for catheter insertion.

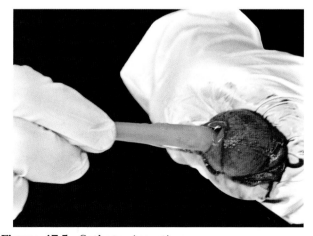

Figure 47-5. Catheter insertion.

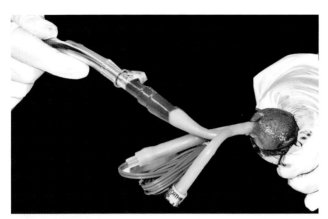

Figure 47-6. Urinary catheter in place attached to closed urinary drainage system.

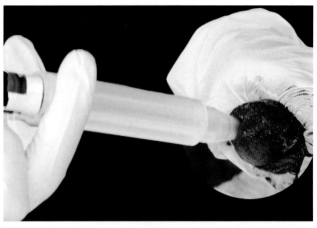

Figure 47-7. Lubricant injected into urethra.

—After urine has drained from the catheter, the balloon should be inflated.

—If the foreskin has been retracted, it should be reduced to anatomical position following successful catheterization.

—The catheter is attached to a closed drainage system (Figure 47-6) and the drainage bag is positioned below the level of the bladder to prevent urinary reflux into the bladder.

■Complications:

—Urethral trauma

—Infection

 Clinical Pearls and Pitfalls

■When catheter passage is difficult, this may be due to one of several problems, including:

—Meatal stenosis

—Urethral stricture

—Prostatic hypertrophy

■Stenoses or strictures may be managed by passage of a smaller catheter.

■Patients with prostatic hypertrophy may be successfully catheterized with a larger catheter or a Coude tipped catheter (which has a stiffer, asymmetric tip).

■The urethra can be distended and lubricated with a lubricant when passage is difficult (Figure 47-7).

■If no urine drains from the catheter after insertion to an appropriate length, the catheter may be irrigated with sterile saline—free saline return suggests that the tip is in the right location.

 Suggested Reading

Thomsen TW, Setnik GS. Male urethral catheterization. *N Engl J Med.* 2006;354:e22.

Wong ES, Hooton TM. Guideline for prevention of catheter-associated urinary tract infections. Center for Disease Control and Prevention Web site. http://www.cdc.gov/ncidod/dhqp/gl_catheter_assoc.html. (Accessed in May 2008.)

CHAPTER 48

Female Urinary Drainage Catheter

 Introduction

Urinary catheter insertion is performed to drain urine from the bladder (Figure 48-1) in patients who are incontinent or have urinary obstruction or to frequently monitor urine output as a proxy for renal function. Long-term catheterization is associated with increased risk of urinary tract infection.

 Definitions and Terms

- French (Fr): The unit of measurement used in sizing urinary catheters—where 1 French equals 1/3 of a millimeter.

- Intermittent straight catheterization: A technique used for intermittent bladder drainage wherein the catheter is inserted and removed periodically to decompress bladder.

 Techniques

- Indications:
  - —Perioperative urinary drainage
  - —Urinary tract outflow obstruction
  - —Urinary volume measurement in the intensive care unit (ICU)

- Contraindications:
  - —Urethral disruption

- Method:
  - —Prior to urinary catheterization, patient consent should be obtained, the urethra and surrounding areas prepped and draped (Figure 48-2), and the universal protocol should be performed as described in Section I.
  - —Prior to catheterization, the operator should wash hands and wear sterile gloves.

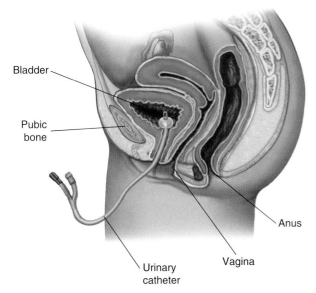

Figure 48-1. Female urinary anatomy.

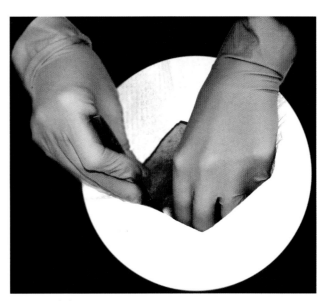

Figure 48-2. Patient preparation.

—According to Centers for Disease Control guidelines:

- Catheters should only be inserted by trained personnel.

- Catheters should only be inserted when necessary, rather than for the convenience of patient-care personnel, and should only be left in place as long as necessary.

- Alternative methods of urinary drainage should be entertained (ie, condom catheter, suprapubic drain).

—The smallest appropriate catheter should be selected for insertion, and the balloon checked for patency.

- Medium catheters (16-18 Fr) are typically used in adult females.

- Larger catheters (20-24 Fr) may be used in patients with hematuria.

—The labia should be spread, the urethra identified, and the catheter should be lubricated and inserted into the urethra (Figure 48-3).

—After urine has drained from the catheter, the balloon should be inflated.

—The catheter is attached to a closed drainage system and the drainage bag is positioned below the level of the bladder to prevent urinary reflux into the bladder.

- Complications:

—Urethral trauma

—Infection

 Clinical Pearls and Pitfalls

- Urethral identification may be difficult in obese patients, patients with prior surgery, following childbirth or with prolapsed of vagina and/or urethra.

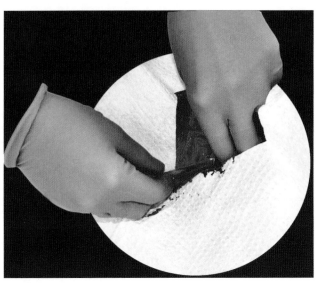

Figure 48-3. Catheter insertion.

- If no urine drains from the catheter after insertion to an appropriate length, the catheter may be irrigated with sterile saline—free saline return suggests that the tip is in the right location.

 Suggested Reading

Leone M. Garnier F. Avidan M. Martin C. Catheter-associated urinary tract infections in intensive care units. *Microbes Infect.* 2004;6:1026–1032.

Wong ES, Hooton TM. Guideline for prevention of catheter-associated urinary tract infections. Center for Disease Control and Prevention Web site. http://www.cdc.gov/ncidod/dhqp/gl_catheter_assoc.html. (Accessed in May 2008.)

CHAPTER 49

Suprapubic Catheterization

 ## Introduction

Suprapubic catheterization is performed as an alternative approach to urinary drainage in patients for whom standard urinary drainage catheters are contraindicated.

 ## Definitions and Terms

- Suprapubic catheter: A catheter inserted into the bladder through the anterior abdominal wall (Figure 49-1).
- Phimosis: Constriction of the foreskin of the penis.

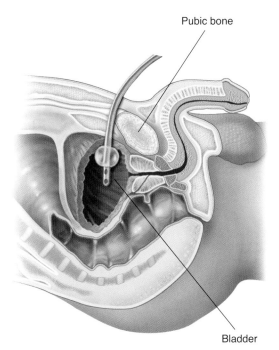

Pubic bone

Bladder

Figure 49-1. Anatomic placement of a suprapubic catheter.

 ## Techniques

- Indications:
  - —Phimosis
  - —Urethral stricture
  - —Chronic urethral infection
- Contraindications:
  - —Coagulopathy
  - —Infected skin over proposed cannulation site
  - —Intra-abdominal pathology (ie, peritonitis, scarring, wound)
  - —Bladder tumor
- Prior to urinary catheterization, patient consent should be obtained, the urethra and surrounding areas prepped and draped, and the universal protocol performed as described in Section I.
- Ultrasound and/or physical examination should be used to identify the location of the bladder.
- Local anesthetic should be infiltrated into the skin over the proposed insertion site.
- A small bore needle or Angiocath is inserted into the bladder and aspirated.
- Aspiration of urine indication successful bladder cannulation and a urinary drainage catheter can be inserted using Seldinger technique or a peel-away introducer sheath.
- Complications:
  - —Bowel perforation
  - —Bladder injury
  - —Hematuria
  - —Infection

 ## Clinical Pearls and Pitfalls

- Failure to aspirate urine following several attempts suggests aberrant anatomy and the procedure should be abandoned in favor of alternative approaches.

▪Suprapubic catheters, while more invasive, may be associated with lower rates of infections.

Suggested Reading

O'Kelly TJ, Mathew A, Ross S, Munro A. Optimum method for urinary drainage in major abdominal surgery: a prospective randomized trial of suprapubic versus urethral catheterization. *Br J Surg.* 1995;82: 1367–1368.

Sethia KK, Selkon JB, Berry AR, Turner CM, Kettlewell MG, Gough MH. Prospective randomized controlled trial of urethral versus suprapubic catheterization. *Br J Surg.* 1987;74:624–625.

CHAPTER 50

Continuous Renal Replacement Therapies

 ## Introduction

Continuous renal replacement therapies have come into increasing use in intensive care units (ICUs), and a variety of alternatives are available, ranging from fluid-removal approaches to continuous dialysis.

 ## Definition and Terms

- Dialysis: Removal of waste products and fluid from the blood.
- Ultrafiltration: Removal of excess fluid from the blood.
- Convection: Movement of solutes and fluid across a semipermeable membrane across which there is a pressure gradient—effective for removal of fluid and certain molecules.
- Diffusion: Movement of (typically small) solutes (like urea) along a concentration gradient from an area of high concentration (the blood) into an area of low concentration (the dialysate).
- Continuous venovenous hemofiltration (CVVH): Convective dialysis which is very efficient at fluid and cytokine removal (Figure 50-1).

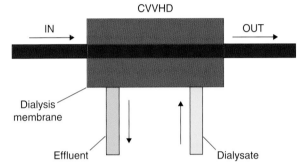

Figure 50-2. CVVHD circuit showing countercurrent dialysis fluid flow relative to blood flow.

- Continuous venovenous hemodialysis (CVVHD): Diffusive dialysis where the dialysate runs "countercurrent" to the blood (Figure 50-2).
- Continuous venovenous hemodiafiltration (CVVHDF): Combination of convective and diffusive dialysis which is common in the ICU and very effective at fluid and solute removal (Figure 50-3).

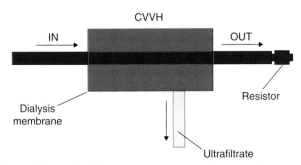

Figure 50-1. CVVH circuit showing the use of an outflow resistor to modify the pressure gradient across the membrane.

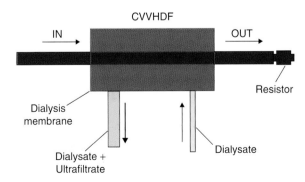

Figure 50-3. CVVHDF circuit showing the combined use of a resistor and countercurrent dialysis to remove fluid and soluted.

■ Continuous arteriovenous hemodialysis: A largely archaic method of continuous dialysis in which arterial blood is processed prior to being reinfused into a vein.

 ## Techniques

■ Prior to initiation of continuous venous dialysis, a special double lumen catheter is placed in a central vein.

■ Vascular cannulation is performed as per the chapter on central line placement (Chapter 34) with the exception that a larger specialty catheter is placed in the vein (Figures 50-4 to 50-7).

■ One lumen of the dialysis catheter is treated as the arterial lumen, for flow proceeding from patient into dialysis machine, whereas the second "venous" lumen is used to return blood to the patient (Figure 50-8).

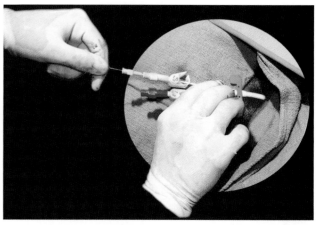

Figure 50-6. Catheter threaded into internal jugular vein.

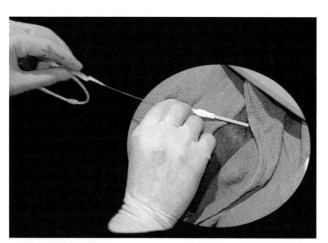

Figure 50-4. Insertion of a large bore dilator over a wire in a Seldinger exchange.

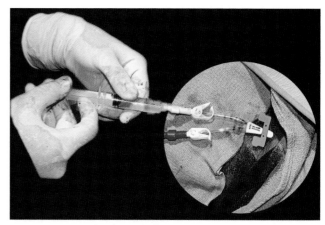

Figure 50-7. Venous lumen injected with heparin flush solution.

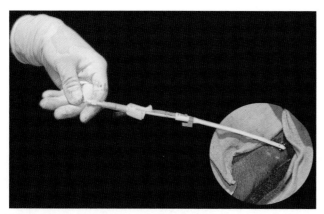

Figure 50-5. Insertion of a double lumen dialysis catheter and dilator over wire.

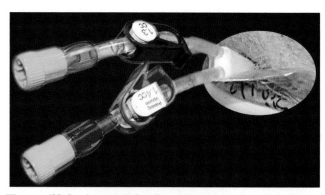

Figure 50-8. Arterial (red) and venous (blue) lumens.

■ Blood is routed through a dialysis machine and the selected dialytic method applied (Figure 50-9).

■ The effluent (equivalent of urine) is measured in the medical record (Figure 50-10).

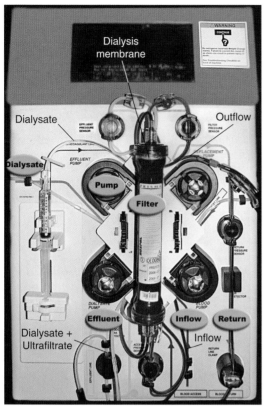

Figure 50-9. Dialysis machine labeled with circuit elements.

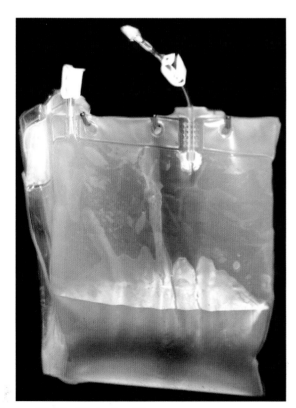

Figure 50-10. Dialysis effluent.

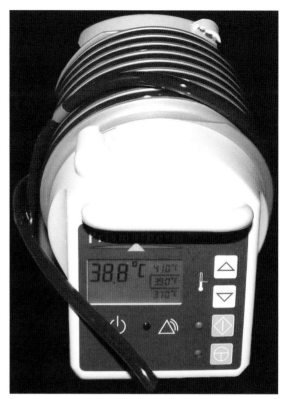

Figure 50-11. Dialysis heater.

▪Blood running through the system is often heated to prevent (Figure 50-11) patient cooling.

 Clinical Pearls and Pitfalls

▪Because critically ill patients are often hemodynamically unstable, a fluid management strategy is essential to prevent excess or insufficient fluid removal.

▪Continuous fluid removal may permit full protein nutrition in patients who would otherwise not tolerate the volume load.

▪Continuous renal replacement therapies may have an effect as an adjuvant in the treatment of sepsis through cytokine removal.

▪Systemic or local anticoagulation is required in continuous renal replacement therapies.

 Suggested Reading

Hall, NA, Fox, AJ. Renal replacement therapies in critical care. *Contin Educ Anaesth Crit Care Pain.* 2006;6:197–202.

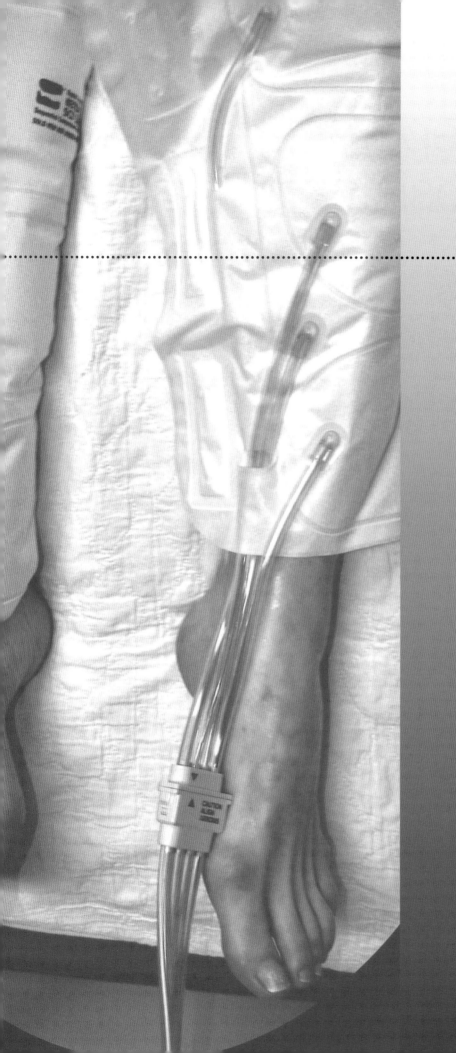

SECTION VII

Extremity Procedures

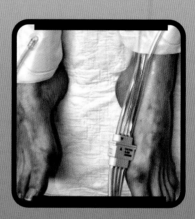

CHAPTER 51

Deep Venous Thrombosis Prophylaxis

 ## Introduction

Deep venous thrombosis (DVT) is a common problem in the ICU. Preventative measures include pharmaceutical and physical measures, the latter of which will be covered in this chapter.

 ## Definitions and Terms

- DVT: Thrombosis in the deep veins of the legs

 ## Techniques

- Sequential compression devices are applied to the calf or calves in bed-bound critically ill patients (Figure 51-1).

 ## Clinical Pearls and Pitfalls

- There is some evidence suggesting that sequential compression devices have antithrombotic effects by acting to inhibit the clotting cascade, so that a single sticking may be worn if there is a contraindication to placement on one leg (ie, vascular surgery).

 ## Suggested Reading

Ramos J, Perrotta C, Badariotti G, Berenstein G. Interventions for preventing venous thromboembolism in adults undergoing knee arthroscopy. *Cochrane Database of Syst Rev.* 2007;(2):CD005259.

Brady D, Raingruber B, Peterson J, et al. The use of knee-length versus thigh-length compression stockings and sequential compression devices. *Crit Care Nurs Q.* 2007;30:255–262.

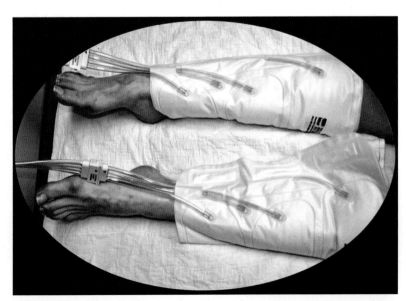

Figure 51-1. Sequential compression devices applied to both ankles.

CHAPTER 52

Diagnosis of Compartment Syndrome

Introduction

Compartment syndrome is an acute process wherein increased pressure in a muscle compartment with a confining fascial compartment leads to ischemia, muscle and nerve damage.

Definitions and Terms

- Interstitial pressure: The pressure in the tissue (typically muscle) in a compartment

Techniques

- Indications for testing:
  —Crush injury
  —Bone fracture
  —Vascular injury
  —Hemorrhage
  —Burns
  —Extravasation of drug or intravenous fluid infusion into compartment
  —Envenomation
  —Excess exercise (ie, running, marching)
  —Casting (ie, after fracture)
- Method:
  —Insert needle attached to transducer into compartment(s) of interest using ad hoc (Figure 52-1) or commercial (Figure 52-2) monitor.
  —Ultrasound may be used to evaluate arterial inflow into a compartment as an adjunct test.
- Tissue pressure greater than 45 mm Hg or within 30 mm Hg of diastolic blood pressure, when accompanied by signs or symptoms of compartment syndrome (ie, pain, paresthesia, weakness, palpable compartment rigidity), is consistent with compartment syndrome and warrants consideration of fasciotomy.

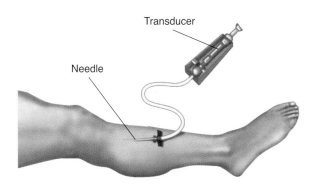
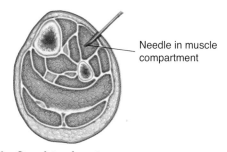

Figure 52-1. Graphic showing compartment measurement using an ad hoc setup.

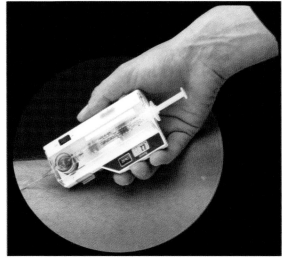

Figure 52-2. Compartment pressure measurement with a commercial tonometer.

Clinical Pearls and Pitfalls

- A high index of suspicion should be maintained in unconscious patients in correct setting and compartment pressure monitored particularly in at-risk compartments in the limbs.

 ## Suggested Reading

Kostler W, Strohm PC, Sudkamp NP. Acute compartment syndrome of the limb. *Injury*. 2005;36: 992–998.

CHAPTER 53

Doppler Evaluation of Pulses

 ## Introduction

Certain patients in the intensive care unit (ICU) are at risk for arterial insufficiency due to arterial injury (ie, aortic or other vascular dissection) or vascular surgery. Portable Doppler evaluation may also be used as an adjunct to standard blood pressure measurement or pulse detection.

 ## Definitions and Terms

Doppler ultrasound: The use of an ultrasound probe and speaker to applied over a vessel to detect flow beneath the probe

 ## Techniques

The tip of the ultrasound probe is lubricated with ultrasonic gel and applied to the skin over vessels in the extremity to detect flow in arteries of interest, such as the *dorsalis pedis* (Figure 53-1) and *posterior tibial* (Figure 53-2) arteries.

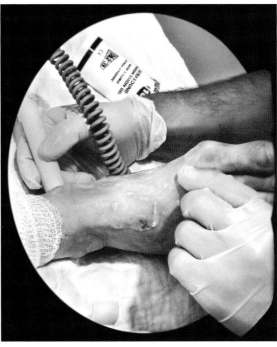

Figure 53-2. Doppler examination of posterior tibial pulse.

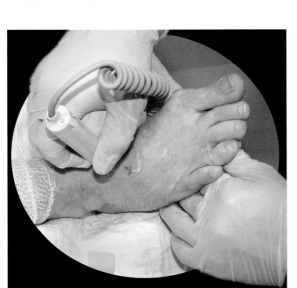

Figure 53-1. Doppler examination of dorsalis pedis pulse.

 ## Clinical Pearls and Pitfalls

If arterial sounds are absent over suspect arteries, the probe should be applied to arteries with pulsatile flow elsewhere on the patient, or the operator may apply the probe to one of his own arteries to verify correct functioning of the device.

 ## Suggested Reading

Campbell WB, Fletcher EL, Hands LJ. Assessment of the distal lower limb arteries: a comparison of arteriography and Doppler ultrasound. *Ann R Coll Surg Engl.* 1986;68:37–39.

CHAPTER 54

Extremity Splinting

 Introduction

Intensive care patients who suffer prolonged immobilization are at risk for development of contractures, and at-risk extremities should be splinted to retain function.

 Definitions and Terms

- Contracture: Muscle and tendon shortening following prolonged disuse

 Techniques

- Resting splints are applied to the hands, wrists, and ankles (Figures 54-1 to 54-5) of intensive care unit (ICU) patients who are unconscious or unable to move for prolonged periods.

 Clinical Pearls and Pitfalls

- Despite the fact that there are little published data showing evidence for the efficacy of splints, many physical therapists advocate their use.

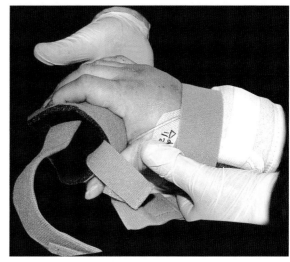

Figure 54-2. Wrist splint applied.

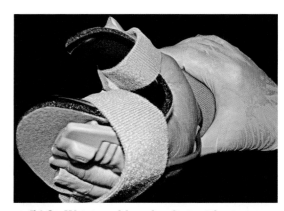

Figure 54-3. Wrist and hand splint with straps.

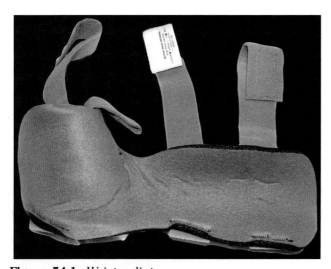

Figure 54-1. Wrist splint.

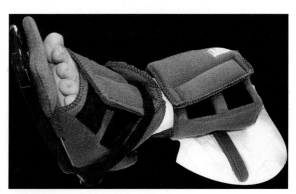

Figure 54-4. Ankle splint.

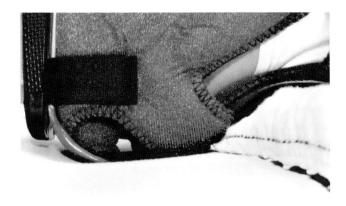

Figure 54-5. Ankle splint showing heel clearance.

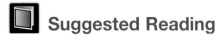 **Suggested Reading**

Stiller K. Physiotherapy in intensive care: towards an evidence-based practice. *Chest.* 2000;118:1801–1823.

CHAPTER 55

Blood Culturing

Introduction

Fever and sepsis work-ups are a routine part of intensive care unit (ICU) care and particularly challenging due to indwelling catheters, and the lack of veins in chronically critically ill patients.

Definitions and Terms

- Aerobic media: Culture media specifically designed to support the growth of aerobic media (Figure 55-1)
- Anaerobic media: Culture media specifically designed to support the growth of anaerobic organisms (Figure 55-1)

Techniques

- A peripheral vein is identified and the skin prepped with a topical disinfectant such as chlorhexidine or povidine-iodine (Figure 55-2).

- The operator should wear sterile gloves if a skin-touch technique is to be used, nonsterile gloves may be used with a no-touch technique (Figure 55-3).
- At least 20 cc of blood should be withdrawn from the site if feasible, and 10 cc injected into both the aerobic and anaerobic media (Figure 55-4).

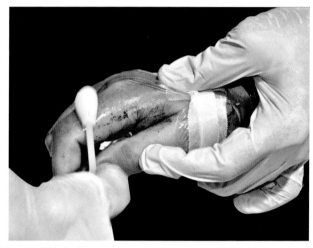

Figure 55-2. Skin preparation.

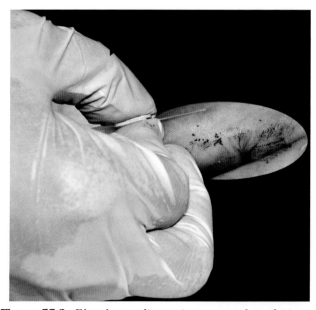

Figure 55-3. Blood sampling using no-touch technique.

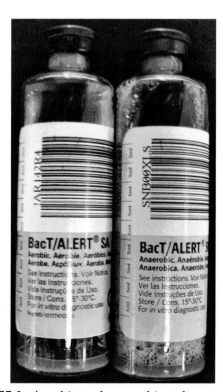

Figure 55-1. Aerobic and anaerobic culture media.

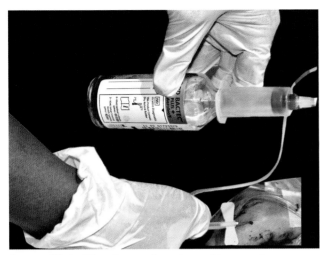

Figure 55-4. Blood sample injected into culture media.

 Clinical Pearls and Pitfalls

Many experts recommend against the practice of drawing blood cultures through existing, indwelling catheters, believing that catheter contamination without true patient infection may lead to false-positive results.

 Suggested Reading

Bates DW, Sands K, Miller E, et al. Predicting bacteremia in patients with sepsis syndrome. *J Infect Dis*. 1997;176: 1538–1551.

Shafazand S, Weinacker AB. Blood cultures in the critical care unit: improving utilization and yield. *Chest*. 2002;122:1727–1736.

Index